Building the Successful Veterinary Practice

VOLUME 3

Innovation and Creativity

Thomas E. Catanzaro
DVM, MHA, FACHE
Diplomate, American College of Healthcare Executives

Iowa State University Press / Ames

Thomas E. Catanzaro, DVM, MHA, FACHE, Diplomate, American College of Healthcare Executives, received his DVM from Colorado State University and his master's in healthcare administration from Baylor University. He was the first veterinarian to receive Board certification with the American College of Healthcare Executives. In the last decade Catanzaro, the author of numerous articles, has visited, assisted, or consulted with over 1,200 veterinary practices in the United States, Canada, and Japan.

© 1998 Iowa State University Press, Ames, Iowa 50014
All rights reserved

Orders: 1-800-862-6657   Fax: 1-515-292-3348
Office: 1-515-292-0140   Web site: www.isupress.edu

Authorization to photocopy items for internal or personal use, or the internal or personal use of specific clients, is granted by Iowa State University Press, provided that the base fee of $.10 per copy is paid directly to the Copyright Clearance Center, 222 Rosewood Drive, Danvers, MA 01923. For those organizations that have been granted a photocopy license by CCC, a separate system of payments has been arranged. The fee code for users of the Transactional Reporting Service is 0-8138-2984-4/98 $.10.

♾ Printed on acid-free paper in the United States of America

First edition, 1998

International Standard Book Number 0-8138-2984-4

Building the Successful Veterinary Practice. Volume 3, Innovation and Creativity

        The Library of Congress has cataloged Volume 1 as follows:

Catanzaro, Thomas E.
    Building the successful veterinary practice: leadership tools. /
Thomas E. Catanzaro. —1st ed.
        p.   cm.
    Includes bibliographical references (p.   ).
    ISBN 0-8138-2819-8
    1. Leadership. 2. Veterinary medicine—Practice.   I. Title.
SF760.L43C37 1997
636.089′068′4—dc21   97-374

Last digit is the print number: 9 8 7 6 5 4 3 2

CONTENTS

PREFACE

Volume 1 explains how to build your practice with leadership skills, from the foundation to the roof. Many of my observations were made while I was building practices and moving my family from one location to another. Later, as Hospital Services Director for the American Animal Hospital Association (AAHA), I helped build a consulting team through which I learned about the application of leadership skills. Also, in Volume 1, I thanked Dick Harder, FACHE, for his healthcare executive mentorship during my Baylor MHA program. Dick also influenced Volume 3, since he now does creativity training for healthcare organizations.

Volume 2 provides the programs and procedures needed by most practices, the furnishings of the house built in Volume 1. Many of these furnishings were created from challenges posed to me by Karyn Gavzer, past marketing director of the American Veterinary Medical Association (AVMA), and Mike Sollars, editor of *Veterinary Forum.* The consulting team of Catanzaro & Associates, Inc., gave me feedback and opinions about the programs and procedures that make a furnished house complete. Also, Rob Deegan had a very special role in Chapter 5 of Volume 2.

Volume 3 is dedicated to the clients of Catanzaro & Associates and to other professional consultants of this profession, like Dr. Ross Clark, Dr. Brent Calhoun, Dr. Dennis McCurnin, Dr. Ray Russell, Don Dooley, and Owen McCafferty, CPA. Thanks to their efforts, and those of respected consultants, writers, and speakers, like Dr. Jack Mara, Bob Levoy, and Dr. Marty Becker, it became evident that traditional leadership skills needed updating. In other books, old management gimmicks were being perpetuated, sometimes with a fancier dressing or a unique twist; which ones are still useful depends upon the people in veterinary practices. Roger Cummings, senior consultant, 1995–1996, was instrumental in helping our consulting team understand this concept from a manager's perspective.

The innovation and creativity of staff members in the many practices Catanzaro & Associates supports clearly show that the hospital director's leadership and accountability make the difference in most every practice.

As a reader and user of all three volumes, you now have the ability to fix a practice "breakdown" and still find a new route to success:

• Volume 1 is the tool kit for building the veterinary practice vehicle.
• Volume 2 is the actual construction of the vehicle to your specifications.
• Volume 3 is the road rally to remember for many days to come.

It is the dedication and professionalism I've seen in hundreds of practices that makes me believe your staff can be successful. Free their minds and take off the restraints of tradition—let innovation and creativity blossom.

Building the Successful
Veterinary Practice

IT HAS TAKEN most veterinarians over 20 years of formal education to learn how to color inside the lines. But before their formal education, during the preschool years, most of them could see entire stories in the clouds and colored outside the lines. Current literature reports that by the time children reach seven years of age, their preschool creativity is reduced by 70 percent. By the time students graduate from veterinary school, there is only one correct answer for each problem (as illustrated by both the National and State Board Examination processes).

The three volumes of *Building a Successful Veterinary Practice* explain how to use leadership to make traditional and time-proven management principles work within the modern veterinary practice. Volume 1, *Leadership Tools,* presents the skills, traits, and philosophies of leadership development. Volume 2, *Programs and Procedures,* applies the skills and principles of leadership development to specific programs within your veterinary practice and life. With this volume, *Innovation and Creativity,* you will remember how to color over and outside the lines. In other words, Volume 1 gives you a tool kit (leadership tools), Volume 2 gives you the skills and knowledge to build the car of your dreams (programs and procedures), and Volume 3 (innovation and creativity) takes you on a new adventure, the road rally, and if you break down, you will have tools to repair your vehicle and get on with your adventure.

This volume may ask you to invite a stranger to have lunch with you, to sing in a crowded elevator, to read Dr. Seuss as a reference text (e.g., *Oh, The Places You'll Go!*), or, worse, to actively listen to other people *before* choosing a course of action. To see if you are ready, please do the following exercise before reading any further:

1. Get the Yellow Pages from the phone book (do it now, we'll wait).

2. Turn to the restaurant listing (again, do it now, we will wait).

3. Count down to the seventh facility listed, and if you have never been there, copy down the name and address. If you have been to the restaurant, choose the next one in the listing that you have never visited (do it, please).

4. Call the restaurant immediately and ensure it is open for dinner tomorrow night (the specific time is not important).

5. Reread number 4 and do it now.

6. Call a friend or a local relative whom you have not seen in over four months *and without any other explanation, invite this person to be your guest for dinner tomorrow night to celebrate his or her recent accomplishment.* Offer no other explanation except to repeat, *"I just heard and want to take you out to celebrate."*

7. Take your guest to the restaurant selected in step 3. Have fun. Don't talk about the office, practice, or business worries. Keep it positive and happy.

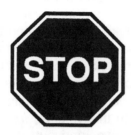

Now, if you read on without completing steps 1 through 7, reference to this exercise will make no sense to you later. This is your chance to be impulsive, innovative, and creative without the fear of failure so common in our veterinary profession. Be adventurous. *Please do the seven steps before reading further.*

You will be asked to do other chores as you breeze through this volume, such as fill in the icebergs with your "thought of the page." In the first two volumes of *Building the Successful Veterinary Practice,* you are given a thought in an iceberg, but on this adventure, you will write the thought you want to retain from the text. In the business world, most every person who reaches the top of his or her profession has written goals. Writing in the iceberg does not guarantee that your practice will be in the top 10 percent, but not doing so will make the chances of your reaching the top slim to none. Remember the 14 leadership skills from Volume 1, and the knowledge-skills-attitude relationship that the iceberg represents.

Volumes 1 and 2 discuss in depth the need to hire for attitude and to commit to an ongoing program of training to a level of trust to build the appropriate skills and knowledge of each team member. When striving for a successful veterinary practice, remember to build with FLAIR:

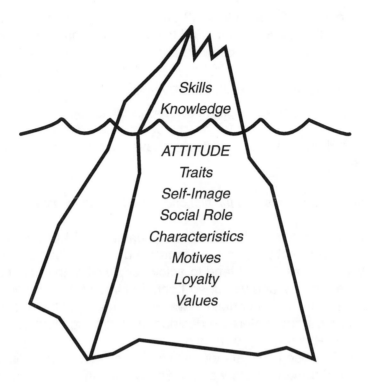

Inside the iceberg:

Skills
Knowledge

ATTITUDE
Traits
Self-Image
Social Role
Characteristics
Motives
Loyalty
Values

Fun is part of the foundation (If you're stuck, you may need more than a jackhammer to free yourself.)

Logic is illogical to lovers (Clients make decisions based on feelings, not logic.)

Accept the unacceptable (When an idea appears inappropriate, just require a 90-day implementation test before evaluating it. There is a natural death rate for poor ideas.)

Innovation is disruptive (The sod house of the frontier prairie was functional in its time, but change results in new designs. Whether you do the unusual as if it were usual, or the usual as if it were unusual, you will be remembered.)

Regardless of the unique design, you must build according to code (The core values of the practice philosophy must not be violated by the leader or the team.)

What does FLAIR mean to you? Let's look at a few real world applications of FLAIR to better understand this change management concept. You may have seen the following printed on Alaskan T-shirts:

The lead dog gets the best views. The rest of the dogs have a view that never changes (it can be called "butt ugly").

Some of those Alaskan T-shirts may have another message on the back (with the appropriate picture):

But the lead dog is also the first one to fall through the hole in the ice!

Across the road from the Medicine Mountain Scout Camp in the Black Hills of South Dakota was a person reputed to be unique and weird. His name was Korczak. Now, I tend to enjoy people who an entire community identifies as unique and weird, so I sought him out. He was where I was told he would be: on a mountain. It was the same area Custer surveyed after the Civil War and before he decided the Little Big Horn Valley was no great threat—but that's another story.

Korczak had been on that mountain three decades—approximately from the time he'd turned 40. He was on his own quest, carried by a vision he was systematically manifesting on that mountain. He knew what he was doing. He was moving rock—blasting tons of it off the mountaintop.

I came wearing my Boy Scout leader's uniform and was allowed into his presence. And there, on that mountain, he shared his vision with me of a 500-foot-tall, over 600-foot-wide great Sioux warrior named Crazy Horse. It was interesting that he knew he would not see the completion of his life's work on that mountain and, at best, his kids might finish the work in their lifetime.

Korczak Ziolkowski died in the early 1980s with the realization of his vision incomplete.

In 1995, I returned to Medicine Mountain Scout Camp to staff a leadership course. I revisited the mountain to see what had become of his life's desire. There were the kids, still blasting and moving rock. They still honored the Scout uniform and allowed us Scout visitors in without charging the nominal admission fee used to subsidize the creation of the colossal sculpture. They said Crazy Horse will be 563 feet high and 641 feet wide and that you could fit the rest of the Mount Rushmore sculpture under his headdress.

They have accepted Korczak's vision.

Most all of us know that Babe Ruth struck out more times than he hit home runs; it's part of his legend. But fewer people know that when Reggie Jackson retired with 563 home runs after 21 major league seasons of professional baseball it put him in the top 10 home run hitters of all time. Interestingly, Reggie struck out 2,597 times and was number one on the major league strikeout record list; the next closest guy had over 600 fewer strikeouts (and about 90 fewer home runs).

When a player is batting .500, it is considered a fluke, but it means 50 percent of the time the player is a loser. What is far more surprising is that with a .300 batting average a player can demand top dollars; it also means this player is failing about 70 percent of the time. In human healthcare, where statistically valid data are kept on relational database mainframe computers, almost 60 percent of new ideas fail, and half of those that don't must be adjusted within the implementation phase just to survive to 90 days.

We veterinarians want gimmicks guaranteed to save our practices. When are we ever going to learn that fear of failure is our greatest enemy?

When I was doing my graduate study at Montana State University, I rented a house with Jim VanDyke (after moving out of a rooming house, eliminating nasty roommates more than once, and living in another house that burned down). Jim and I had a relationship that went back over three years, to when we were required to room in the dorm unless we pledged a fraternity, which Jim and I did to get out of the dorm, but that is another story. This is the story of the great preowned sofa we bought for $15.

We had rented the house and needed furniture and found the sofa in a preowned furniture store (back then it was called a secondhand store). I am about six foot tall and Jim was taller than me by a few inches; the one-piece, nine-foot-long sofa had one-foot-wide arms, great for sitting on at a party, and a seven-foot seating area, great for stretching out on. The $15 cash-and-carry deal was too good to pass up. The challenge was getting it into the living room. There was a small, tight-left-hand-turn vestibule at the front door, and the sofa would not make the angle. We could get it through the back door, into my bedroom, in a straight shot, but then the fun began. The route from the bedroom door, into the hallway, then into the living room was another tight right-hand turn, and the nine-foot sofa would not bend. We looked for an alternative.

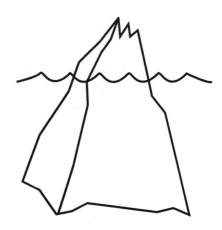

The answer was not hard for two college guys. Remove the sofa legs and the bedroom doorjamb to take the sofa into the hallway and then angle it upward through the bedroom door, standing it up on end in the hallway. This only meant we had to put one hole in the ceiling of the hallway, into the attic, since the ceilings were just under nine foot. This allowed us to angle it up then twist it and angle it back down into the living room. After reinstalling the legs, we were ready to rock and roll. The ceiling was not that hard to patch, and we could reattach the doorjamb anytime. We just knew what we had to do, and we did it. When we had to move out because the house was condemned, we waited until the front wall was removed, walked back in, and took the sofa out the hole in the wall.

Now my wife of 30-plus years makes me measure doors and angles before we shop for furniture. This represents the learning curve of marriage: "Don't make a mess" and the sequel "Clean up after yourself, now!" In short, like the first grader who is now proud of coloring inside the lines, I have been trained to a household standard—*do not remove walls or ceilings.* (People who have known us during our long years of wedded bliss call my wife Saint Anne for what she has put up with, like our 17 moves in the first 21 years of marriage.)

When I departed the American Animal Hospital Association (AAHA) in 1991, after the lawyers decided consulting was too great a liability to the hospital if it offered solutions, I needed an office. I also needed low rent and lower overhead, since I was going to "income finance" Catanzaro & Associates, Inc., into existence. I went on a quest for appropriate space and found Heritage Square, an amusement park built as the Disneyland of Denver in the early 1960s that went into receivership during the mid-1980s oil crisis and emerged with a very limited number of Main Street retail shops and a mountainside alpine slide surrounded by a kiddy ride activity area. The back street had remained generally unoccupied since Heritage Square had reopened from receivership. My mentors, many from AAHA, strongly suggested I reconsider the location, since an amusement park was not appropriate for a veterinary consultant image.

Ignoring the conservative warnings, I approached the management office of Heritage Square and was told it only rented to retail merchants. I stated I knew the park had not rented to anyone in the past four years, and the spokesperson stated the policy was to rent only to retail merchants and would not bend from the retail only position. So I rephrased my request as follows: "I need to rent about 1,400 square feet so I can build a training room within the office complex so I can bring people to the Square for training, over the lunch hour, during the winter, when there generally were no tourists in the Square."

The rest is history. Catanzaro & Associates was physically built in Heritage Square by Phil Seibert and myself, to unique facility designs we developed, based on our desires for and knowledge of our operational style. We used a lot of interior glass walls, standing desks (required for veterinarians used to the examination table), and built-in shelves to make the best use of wall space. The Square management found that office rent paid its operational bills better than no rent at all. The back street of Heritage Square now has a sign that states this street is primarily light industry and offices. As we enter our seventh year, we are the old-timers on the back street, and the Square management has kept the occupancy high with alternative tenants.

There was a practice of the living dead. I can't think of anything else to describe the feeling of the practice. The doctors and staff would be animated and outgoing while in the examination room with clients, but as soon as they left the exam room, a no-emotions attitude would come over them. There was no fun, no small talk. They went about their duties as if they were robots. For most of the initial three days on-site, I tried to break down the walls of this zombieville, but I did not make a dent!

Late on the third day, after I announced what I thought the team could do, based on the strengths I had found, one kennel person shared an insight with me. The senior technician had just left the practice a month ago, after a four-year tenure (actually a reign of terror). Her style of management was lurking and listening, then using anything said as a tool for the next attack on people. I don't know if it was vengeful, or innate, but it was destructive. For instance, she had brought in a used condom found around the practice's plow vehicle parking place and dropped it on the owner's desk, stating that she had "found this from his girlfriend-courting area"; how do you object to this type of untruth without sounding defensive? The staff had learned to say nothing, do nothing, or try nothing that she could use against them.

She departed, but the practice owner did not take the leadership to reverse the habits. Oh yes, he had tried staff meetings, but many had excuses for not coming, and those who did sat emotionless and silent. Maybe that was the reason I had been brought in. I had to reverse the process, but I was leaving the site in 60 minutes; what could I do in that short of a time period? I scheduled a return visit, to be done at my cost since I was passing through the area, so I could conduct a special 100 percent attendance evening staff meeting.

The staff meeting was actually a behavior profile session, using the D-I-S-C (domi-

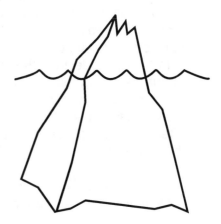

nant, inspirational, steadiness, and conscientious) personal profile system, an instrument far more behavior-based than many of the other personality-profiling tools available (e.g., Myers Briggs). It could also be replicated by the practice leadership without the aid of my team or an outside scoring agency. It is an immediate, individualized, and accurate response and assessment tool for normal and stress response situations. The D-I-S-C was administered to each staff member, and we then discussed why each profile type would be important to an average veterinary practice. After this, we shared each person's profile, using a team-profiling sheet so each person had a written description of each team member's behavior. We then discussed how to approach each behavior profile when under stress, why each profile needed others, and for what aspects, and how the practice could use the profile to increase cooperation. After about 90 minutes, the team members started asking for weekly staff meetings and more feedback opportunities, and more importantly, they were having fun talking about each other's behavior profile. It was now okay to be who they were; it was an accepted strength rather than a weakness.

The first day on-site during any consultation finds me just floating and observing the interactions between staff, clients, and healthcare providers. I was in a practice that was stalled: the owner was burnt out and thought he might need to leave the profession (so what's new, you ask). I handed out the staff opinion surveys and did the 100 medical records audit (see Appendix F) the first evening. On the second morning, I was in the owner's office and asked a question very uncommon for me, specifically, "Why are those two ladies at your front desk?" Sputtering, the owner said, "They were here when I bought the practice. ... I was going to release them last month, but since you were coming, I waited." I asked how things had gotten to where they were and was told, "They knew all the clients and had a great rapport with them." So I rephrased the question: "These two ladies are undermining the protective healthcare program. They tell clients that you will talk about feline leukemia, but it is only a low-incidence problem for cats that live outside, and they probably don't need treatment for it. How can you accept that?"

In short, we decided they needed to be released, but there was a fear about unemployment costs. I stated I was worried about the employment costs to the practice, so we worked out a dehire process. I sat with the hospital manager, outside the practice, and we rehearsed the narrative for the afternoon. I advocate a positive approach to dehiring, and recommended the following:

Call them in on Thursday afternoon and tell them you are worried about them. Tell them they have been valuable members of the team but recently seem unhappy. For this reason, you want to give them "the rest of the week off with pay." You want them to take the time to contemplate their current feelings. Suggest they use the time to see what other employment opportunities are available in the community and at what requirements. Then set the final requirement, "Come back Monday morning with a new attitude, ready to support doc 110 percent, or bring in a resignation. If you bring in a resignation, we will give you your vacation and sick pay, write a good letter of recommendation, and tell positive things to all prospective employers who call. If you come back in and say you will support doc, but revert to the old behavior, you will be released for cause, without a benefit payout, and without a letter of recommendation, and if any prospective employer calls, we will tell that person the truth.

I asked the manager what she would say when they refuted the observation. She started to justify it, but I stopped her and said she could do it with a much shorter response, such as,

See, that is exactly what I am talking about. Your first response is to argue, rather than agreeing and supporting the observation 110 percent. This is exactly what you must self-assess while you are taking the rest of the week off with pay. Leave now and please start thinking about your future role in the practice.

They left and turned in the uniforms and letters of resignation by the following morning. We had a staff luncheon planned for day three and received the most unusual feedback from the rest of the team. They said they wondered how long the owner would tolerate them, that whenever they had to work with them it took them three days to get a positive attitude back. To which the owner asked why they hadn't said anything, and they responded, "They worked for you and we needed to support you, so we did what you asked us to do."

The owner had a revelation that the solution was within him. The replacement process took four months, using a full team interview process. He hired based on competency *and* team fit, without compromise or excuse, promoted feedback and open discussion during the decision process, and tolerated no one who fought the team once a decision was made. With this new team-centered perspective, he grew from one stalled practice to six growing practices in the following 24 months.

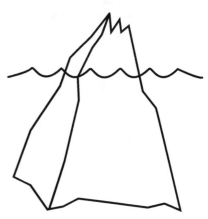

The Road Rally—Design the New Paradigm

When revving up your innovation engine, make sure the engine is tuned, there is adequate fuel, and the garage is ventilated! Do not do this between clients or in the evening when there has been a 12-hour day of crisis. Look at the following three elements required for revving safely when attacking a problem.

Engine tuning

Engine tuning represents defining the problem. You must know how you got where you are, what the community is expecting, and what the feelings are of those around you. All resources must be known and necessary data accumulated (or at least available), you must be aware of your staff's and your own verbal and nonverbal communication skills, and needs must be assessed, from the needs of the one to the needs of the many (thank you Dr. Spock for the phrase). This stage is actually more theory than substance.

1. Issue definition teams should be three to five people.

2. At intervals of 45 minutes, the teams need to be remixed and build off what has gone before or any other resources.

3. Seek quality as well as quantity for best results, but protect all the ideas; no value judgments, please.

Adequate fuel

Adequate fuel represents the initial ideas and visions. The fuel is the potential and must be mixed in the tuned engine of resources. Take into account the characteristics and needs of staff, clients, patients, and primary providers. This stage depends on inspiration.

1. A scribe is often an asset, unless the scribe uses the position to hide or promote a specific agenda—then a scribe is counterproductive.

2. Here the ideas get their octane rating during the reverse side, four-corner, targeted input exercise (see the following section, Index Card Fuel Categorization).

3. Great glee is a capper in each session (cheering, team spirit, applause, etc.). The scribe should ensure everyone feels appreciated and charged before the total group reconvenes.

Ventilated garage

A ventilated garage represents an environment where ideas can be fairly evaluated. The environment should promote idealism, imagination, and open-armed acceptance. This stage depends on everyone considering the practicality, feasibility, and marketability of ideas.

1. Evaluation is generally done within the larger combined group, where the scribes present the best of the best.

2. The teams freely add and embellish as the scribes report to the total group.

3. There is a group leader moderator/recorder using a chart pad to capture the excitement of the additions and embellishments.

4. The finale is the chart pad expansion, where the microscopic evaluations in the final review make the bad worse and the great the "bestest" ever.

Each of the three elements of revving up your innovation engine must be separate activities. Do not let them run into each other or be limited by some outside pressure. If any phase stalls, try a new approach: look at it from a totally different perspective (become an animal looking at the veterinary delivery system); change your position (move locations, change your posture); play different music; let the weird become the normal, and the radical become the average (innovation is disruptive—don't block it); or even take a break and do some mind-altering activity (juggle, cook, play handball, mow the lawn, become active rather than thoughtful for a while). Don't rush the evolution process. Allow at least three hours for each step to evolve and have a two-hour break between each.

Index Card Fuel Categorization

Accumulating adequate fuel can be a challenge at times, especially in a busy veterinary practice. So here is how to develop creative thinking.

1. Keep those resources available from engine tuning and proceed to an off-site location, with at least three hours to kill.

2. Get multiple bundles of 3x5-inch cards (different colors), a big box of Crayolas (or even washable markers if you like the aroma), and abundant supplies of coffee, tea, and high-caffeine soda. Make sure there are toilet facilities and a fresh air source (nothing is worse than stale air when working with fuel).

3. Identify categories for the fuels, based on the project at hand, and give each category its own 3x5 card color. Categories can include community opportunities, practice practicalities, environmental threats, staff limitations, expenses, strong resources, or whatever you think will cause great ideas to flow.

4. Any idea that comes to you or any member of the team, whether it appeals to you or not, gets written on a separate card. State the idea aloud as you think of it so others can get the vibrations of your efforts and then throw the card onto the floor.

5. When the floor is carpeted with ideas, each team member takes turns picking up two cards of different colors and then writing a third idea, an integration of the two ideas, on a card with a color that applies. Keep up the momentum; don't let the process stall.

6. Take a respite from the process when the ideas start slowing and head for a food break—make it last at least an hour.

7. When you return, someone must write something on each of the four back corners of the prime cards (those with ideas that are really exciting for someone on the team), and if no one can, the ideas do not get processed. This is actually the first part of ventilating the garage: getting ready for the culling process. We find that using the four *f*s for this assessment is a good starting point for the corner categories: *f*eelings, *f*acts, *f*un, and *f*inances. *You might have another four perspectives for filling in the corners.* If so, use them. One client has used C-A-R-E: *c*lient, *a*ction, *r*e-

spect, *excellence*. One national franchise we all know and love, McDonald's, was built using Q-V-S-C: *q*uality, *v*alue, *s*ervice, and *c*leanliness.

Start Your Engines

This is where you should return to Volume 1, review the 14 leadership skills, and look at how to apply these within your practice:

Group forming has already been done.
- Knowing and using the resources of the group
- Effective communication
- Understanding the characteristics and needs of the group

The transitional skills have been applied.
- Reflection
- Representing the group

The application elements now come into play.
- Evaluating
- Effective teaching
- Planning
- Internal promotion
- Situational leadership
- Group development
- Personal relationships
- Setting the example
- Continuous quality improvement

The application of these 14 leadership skills requires commitment, personal discipline, and behavior modification. They should have been applied to each program and procedure in Volume 2. Applying these will make the adventure of innovation and creativity easier, and once a caring leader starts to color outside the lines, it will be impossible to go back to demanding performance from the practice team through decrees. Think of some of the common quotes you have heard as they apply to innovation and creativity:

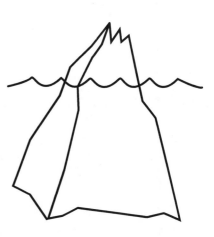

Luck is being prepared to grab opportunity as it passes by.

When you win, nothing hurts!

The will to win is important, but the will to prepare is vital.

It's not over till it's over!

Nothing important was ever achieved without taking a chance.

Chance favors the prepared mind.

It is not the size of a person but rather the size of her heart that matters.

Fortune favors the bold!

Today is the first day of the rest of your life.

May our adversaries make us strong,
may our victories make us wise,
may our actions make us proud.

Application Exercise

Believe it or not, at the end of each chapter, there will be a mind map!

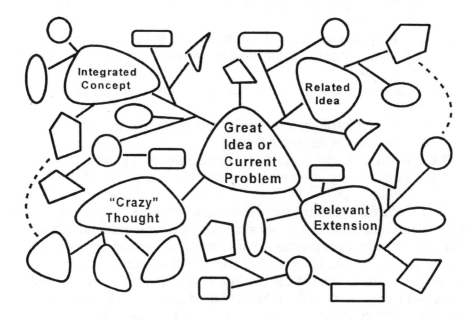

The mind map was conceived in England many years ago by the Learning Methods Group as a research method for promoting brainstorming. About half of people think about key concepts in an interrelated and integrated manner, and the other half break them down into rows and columns. The column-and-row way of thinking works for taking notes in veterinary school, but it doesn't always allow consideration of pros/cons and multiple alternatives. Working out from a core idea suits the brainstorming methodology and offers a way to slot ideas into the core concept without having to highly organize the thought process.

Mind mapping is based on getting as many crazy and wild ideas as possible in the shortest period of time. Write whatever comes into your head; initially quantity, not quality, counts. No value judgments, no criticisms, not even "constructive critiques" are allowed at the beginning. There is plenty of

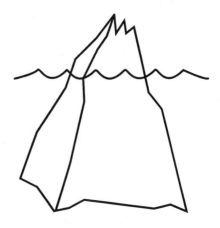

time for these limiting thoughts later! Whenever you write something, build on it; this is called piggybacking (an appropriate term for veterinarians).
Here are some basic steps for the mind-mapping exercise:

- ✐ Write the challenge or core idea in the center of a blank page.
- ✐ Draw a circle around it.
- ✐ Write each major facet at the end of a line from the core issue.
- ✐ Draw lines (roads) outward from each new item and brainstorm for more details.
- ✐ Add branches to lines as necessary and add main roads when indicated.
- ✐ Start to color the lines of thought (roads) with different colors; use one color for ideas in the same flow.
- ✐ Circle main thoughts and/or link related topics with connecting lines.
- ✐ Look again at the mind map for additional interrelationships.

Mind mapping is an excellent technique not only for generating new ideas but also for developing your intuition. Once you get used to the mind map, you can apply the process to anything from business to relationships to your future. To help, at the end of each chapter I have provided the beginnings of a mind map. After you read each chapter, take the iceberg ideas you have added on the odd-numbered pages and expand on the issues identified on the mind map (see the sample on p. 19).

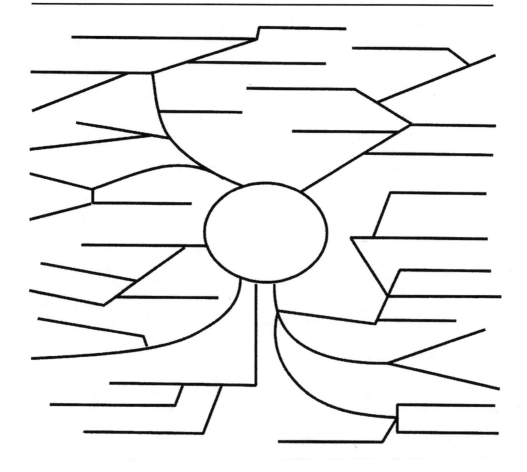

Evolving Perspectives of Veterinary Practice

Entering the New Playing Field

In 1987, Tom Peters wrote *Thriving on Chaos: Handbook for a Management Revolution,* and in 1989, Richard Semelar wrote "Managing without Managers," published in the *Harvard Business Review.* Yet in 1995 we saw articles like *"*Changing the Role of Top Management: Beyond Structure to Processes*"* published in the *Harvard Business Review,* as if we didn't take the hint during the 1980s. The fact is in veterinary medicine the superstores and corporate practices began moving into neighborhoods because *no one* was willing to make the practice culture change needed to meet emerging client needs. Volume 2 of *Building the Successful Veterinary Practice* discusses the "New American Veterinary Practice" as a basis for establishing the programs and procedures needed to thrive in this changing environment. The chaos created by this change can be controlled, but not prevented, if practices are willing to risk chaos in their delivery of healthcare.

Modern veterinary practices will be based on a triad formed by the healthcare provider, the staff, and the client as queen or king. The winners will be competitive, robust, patient advocates, fast, dominant, flexible, adaptable, fun, innovative, and caring. In the next few years, pressures such as alternative providers, the knowledge explosion, litigation, resource scarcity, competitors, market changes, regulations, cost of technology, and uncertainty will require the veterinary practice leader to be:

Client focused
Provides easy access and rapid service-client-response (SCR), de-

creases costs, increases quality factors, removes the negatives, adds to the perceived value, encourages friendly facilities and greater market service, addresses wants and meets needs.

A systems controller

Redesigns jobs, re-engineers functions, streamlines cycle time, leads the benchmarks, has brass tack toughness pursuing values and vision, assigns accountability for outcomes, has solid measurements for outcome expectations, celebrates success.

An associate empowerer

Hires doctors and staff who unilaterally serve the client and improve the system, fosters training and nurturing for individuals and teams, shows respect-recognition-responsibility, maximizes utilization, and encourages freedom.

An uncommon leader

Grows the problem-change-activities (PCA), fits the organization to the users and doers, listens to clients and staff, believes in innovation and creativity, gets results and ideas rather than just status, has a just-do-it (JDI) attitude.

Values driven

Has an effervescent vision, kills problems rather than ideas, encourages fun and celebration, has a bias for action (JDI), welcomes creative chaos, increases speed and adaptability, attacks barriers to change and innovation.

I have added acronyms to the above five factors just to force you to use a new nomenclature in seeking creative approaches to problem resolution. Often, a new vocabulary is the first step in innovation. Leaders also continually examine the relationships within their practices. The interrelations diagram in Figure 1.1 conveys the structure of today's veterinary practice.

The real secret of empowerment is to simply get off the backs of the staff; stop undermining the team. Take down the electric fences put up in the past, those caused by the question "Why did you do *that?*" or the statement "We never did it that way!" Change the typical challenging manager's statement to a leader's question of concern: instead of "Why were you late?" say, "I missed you at 7:00 this morning, is everything okay?" Remember, (1) people have a life outside the practice, (2) no one in healthcare delivery can be an island, and (3) the practice core values are inviolate. Look at the structure of your practice and redefine relationships. Nurture *everyone* to stretch "outside the box" of his or her paradigms.

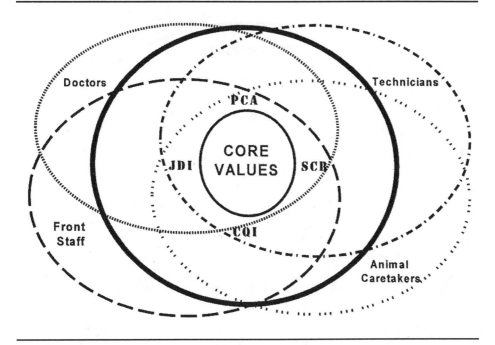

Fig. 1.1. The New American Veterinary Practice organization, version 1.

Ready for a new acronym? B-HAGs (big, hairy, audacious goals). Always remember the vision and mission of the practice. Planning and effective teaching are two critical leadership skills (see Vol. 1, *Building the Successful Veterinary Practice: Leadership Tools*) that will remind staff members of the practice's vision and mission and reinforce the staff's role as patient advocates. These factors—vision, mission, planning, client service, patient advocacy, and effective teaching—are determined by the core values of the practice. This is illustrated by a modification of Figure 1.1 (Fig. 1.2).

Now is a time to look at an innovation for making it happen. A "do it" project (see the DIG Board in Appendix A) for any B-HAG has 60 days to get solved. Warp speed is necessary in change management. If a problem can't be identified and resolved utilizing the available resources in 60 days, it is redefined into smaller pieces that can be. The minimum number of goals for any veterinary practice that desires to excel should be one B-HAG for every staff member every

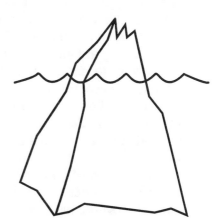

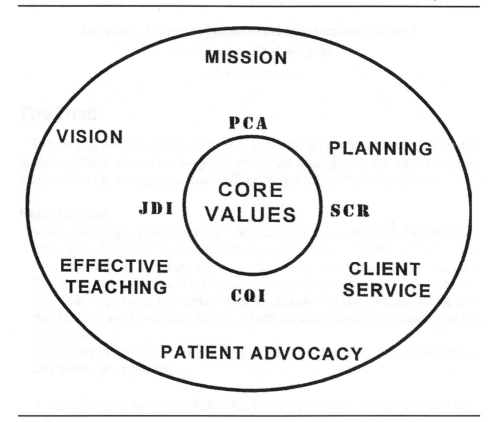

Fig. 1.2. The New American Veterinary Practice organization, version 2.

quarter, with 75 percent staff participation annually. In the first year of the process, there should be monthly B-HAGs, and the staff participation needs to be 75 percent quarterly. The intellectual capital of a practice team is an intangible asset, but like a force field, it is real.

Citibank has estimated its intellectual capital to be three to four times the book value of its business. Consider what a surgical specialty practice did after looking at Figure 1.1. This was a one-owner specialty practice, with two associate surgeons, each keeping 35 percent of the billable fees. It had three revenue flows: a mobile surgical practice, a referral surgical practice, and an in-house surgery practice at the central referral center of the metroplex. Each surgeon had his or her own primary technician ("organizational liaison" was used instead of "supervisor" because of the open work environment). The organization was developed to include a technician liaison and a paraprofessional liaison, as shown in Figure 1.3, by the owner (before our discussion). Then we had our discussion, and the surgeon discovered his technician liaison must also coordinate with the tech-

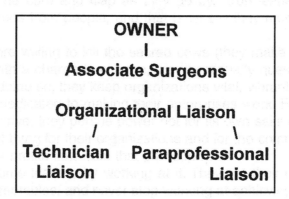

Fig. 1.3. Old surgical practice organization.

nicians at the practices being supported by the mobile unit, and the paraprofessional liaison must take time to train the front teams at those practices on the benefits of using the mobile surgery team. The old line diagram was not viable, but the owner did not know of any others until I showed him the triple-yolk egg picture (Fig. 1.4). On seeing it, his only response was, "Yes, that is it!" He left satisfied, and his team became aware of the spheres of influence it had.

Remember Mother Nature? Look to her for the secrets of innovation and creativity. Human intelligence (HI) emerges from "neural conversation": millions of messages expend energy to develop a thought. In the same way organizational intelligence (OI) is the result of staff and client conversation. Who's got the brain power?

> We dance around in a ring and suppose,
> But the secret sits in the middle and knows.
> —Robert Frost

It is not that a leader does not get great ideas, but a great leader (1) lets the team enhance the ideas until it owns them and (2) creates the environment that nurtures change. The visions and values of the great leaders are centered on client needs and rapid response to those needs (SCR). These leaders encourage conversation and

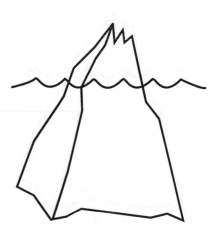

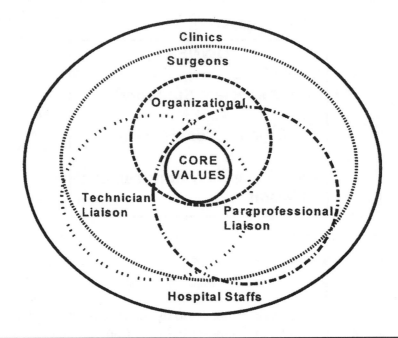

Fig. 1.4. New surgical practice organization.

feedback in this new, open environment, use all the brains available to re-solve a problem (PCA), expect change (JDI), and use creative chaos as the standard to measure innovation and creativity (OI). Consequently, these leaders will foster continuous quality improvement (CQI). Create chaos and you can control it; allow someone else to create it and you can only react to it. The choice is yours!

Barnacles: Practices That Resist Change

The barnacle is confronted with a major decision early in its existence: where it is going to live? Once the decision is made, the barnacle spends the rest of its life with its head cemented to a rock or boat bottom. Not unlike some of the veterinarians we know.

Charles Darwin spent nine years categorizing barnacles. Although he became the recognized authority on these creatures, it slowed his explo-ration of evolution. Despite the peer recognition and fame, Darwin stated his was an imbalanced dedication. Some veterinary practices and practi-tioners stall in midcareer, too. Remember the barnacle.

Hanging in There

We have all seen the pictures of critters desperately hanging on to a branch with the poster caption "hang in there" ... cute, funny, yet in real life disastrous. A practice's commitment to survive is commendable, but survival is seldom progressive to the practice team. A consultant must view such practices with compassion. Assessing the reasons for the hang-in-there mind-set is how an enhancement plan is initiated. Often, the practitioner or practice faced a problem that could not be solved with the available resources, or something or someone inflicted a major wound on the staff's confidence or self-esteem. In some cases, they were pulled down by hidden resentments or family-learned dysfunctions. The feeling of being defeated creeps into everyone's life at some time. Some people become cynical and sour, while others become stubborn and cement to the status quo for security reasons; either reaction is detrimental.

Every practitioner has his or her own vision of practice excellence and success, and that is what the target needs to be. What is categorized as hanging in there in my mind is when a practice culture stops individuals from learning or growing. It may appear busy, but close evaluation reveals the staff just going through the motions. Following established procedures in itself isn't pathogenic. Life is hard. Just to keep going is sometimes a significant act of courage. However, I do worry about women and men who function far below the level of their potential, and I become especially concerned when the development of the individual is retarded by the practice management philosophy or apprehensions.

We must face the fact that many veterinarians out there are more stale than they really know. Just look at the rate of continuing education by themselves or their team members. Often, these veterinarians and staff are more bored than they care to admit. Boredom is a secret ailment of many practices. The boss is so concerned with ensuring process that the outcomes as well as the original reasons for operation are lost in the quest for mediocrity. If boredom can rise to the level of a mystical experience, some of the busiest veterinarians are among the great mystics of our day.

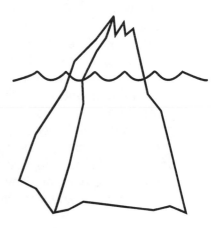

Complacency and Rigidity

We can't write off the dangers of complacency and imprisonment by professional habits and opinions. These are inherent characteristics of any professional who has been taught there is one best way; they are especially ingrained in healthcare professionals because they must be concerned about malpractice and community practice standards. Look around—even at people who are younger than you. Many people are trapped by fixed attitudes and habits. Like a clock with frozen hands, they will occasionally be perfectly right, which will reinforce the validity of their inflexible positions. I've worked within professional veterinary medicine associations and could list "leaders" whose clocks have stopped and could even tell you approximately what year it occurred.

Everything that occurs is actually offering us options; there are many paths. What is important is how a path is followed or, better yet, how someone *leads* a team down or up the path. Leadership is key to making successful choices. Risk is associated with every choice in life, and the failure to take a risk is in fact a risk.

If we are aware that there is a continual danger of mental atrophy, we can initiate countersurveillance measures. Sometimes we hear the complacency: "We have always done it this way." Sometimes we can see it: the mandatory smile when greeting a client. Occasionally you can smell it, as in "I smell an old habit recurring, musty and stagnant." Some veterinarians have fur-lined their ruts so well that they feel change is just not possible for them, that life and their practices have them trapped. This is not fact; it is perception. Life can take unexpected turns.

It is not unlike trappers who trekked across snowcapped mountains with snowshoes and a load of furs. The smart trappers knew which ravines led down to water and shelter, and the adventurous kept trying until they found the way. The less smart didn't explore alternatives below the snowline because this meant they had to take off their snowshoes. Their bones are preserved in the snowfields.

Prisons and Jailers

We seldom build our own prisons. Our society, family life experiences, and parents have had a major hand in building them. These three factors created the roles and self-images that influenced our career choices and held us captive for so long. Any individual who selects a new path in life will have to deal with the ghosts of the past—the memories of earlier failures, the remnants of childhood experiences and revolts, the accumulated resentments that have long outlived their cause. Some people cling to their ghosts with a tenacity that sometimes approaches a form of pleasure but concurrently hampers their growth. As mountain climbers state, "You never conquer the mountain, you only conquer yourself."

Although others may have been instrumental in building our prisons, we are our own jail keepers. We often consider growing up a function of adolescence, but it continues much longer (to those who are parents of teenagers, I apologize for scaring you with this statement). It takes an adult to learn how to release him- or herself from the prison of the past; if it occurs by age 40, you should consider yourself lucky. There is a myth that you can't teach an old dog new tricks; people who work in veterinary medicine knows this is false, but they still put limitations on themselves. It's what you learn after you think you know it all that really counts.

The jail keeper in you must be awakened. Learn from your misadventures; learn from your successes. When you hit a spell of trouble, ask your jail keeper, "What is life trying to teach me?" We learn from families, friends, and life encounters. We learn by suffering, by growing older, and by bearing up under the things we can't change. We learn faster by nurturing others, by loving, and by taking risks. The lessons are not always happy ones, but they keep coming. It isn't bad to occasionally pause and look inward, to challenge that jail keeper inside you, and to reflect on choices ignored or cast away as inappropriate. By midlife, most people have become fugitives from themselves!

Barnacles Are Not on Mountaintops

There are many different type of barnacles, and Charles Darwin identified them. But they all live below the surface, and they don't make waves. They just survive. People scramble up the mountain of life. They sweat and strain to reach a new plateau where they can catch their breath. It is curious that, as we reach each plateau, we depend on others' judgment to learn about our own achievement; it is more curious that most people use scales to rate achievement, such as A-B-C-D-F or 1 to 10.

As you ascend your mountain, you reach some intermediate goals. When you stand on that plateau and look around, chances are there is an empty feeling, maybe even more than just a little empty. You wonder if the climb is worth it or, worse, if you are climbing the wrong mountain. But life isn't a mountain with a single summit; it isn't Curly's single-finger answer to life (as in the movie *City Slickers*); it isn't a game that has a final score. It is an endless unfolding of self-discovery. It is an endless and unpredictable dialogue between potentials and life situations.

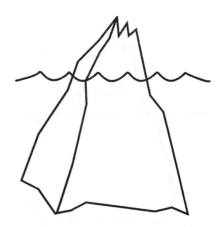

Unlike the barnacle, each person has more resources of energy than he or she has tapped—more talent, more dreams, more strengths than have ever been tested. Each person can give more, given the right environment, the appropriate cause, and the belief it can be done.

Motivation

As people begin to see themselves in a new light, obstacles from their life experiences are replaced by motivation from their inner strengths. Horse sense, the sense horses have not to bet on people, is considered a valuable trait, but as leaders, we must learn to bet on people. That is why it is smarter to hire for attitude and train for the skills than it is to hire for skills and try to develop the attitude. The world is moved by highly motivated people, by enthusiasts, by men and women who want something very much and believe in the adventure of life.

I'm not talking about ambition. Ambition wears out. But a zest for life can continue forever. Most humans cannot achieve the complacency of the barnacle. People are worriers and puzzlers; they want meaning in their lives. As Robert Louis Stevenson said, "Old or young, we're on our last cruise." Meaning is built from the past, the present, and the dreams of what can be. It is based on your specific talents, your love, and the values for which you are willing to make sacrifices. Keep a sense of curiosity, discover new things, care, risk failure, reach out, or, in short, be interested. Remember, your perspective on life will help determine your personal success.

It's a Matter of Perspective

You don't buy coal, you buy heat;
You don't buy circus tickets, you buy thrills;
You don't buy a paper, you buy news;
You don't buy spectacles, you buy vision;
You don't buy a water heater, you buy hot water;
You don't buy printing, you buy selling.
—Anonymous

The perspective of the practice leader sets the tone of practice operations. It is difficult to generalize about leaders because leaders are different in style, approach, and motivation. But one generalization that can be made is that leaders do not lead organizations or corporations; they understand that they lead people. A leader cannot lead unless someone is there to follow, and the best know how to make it exciting.

The man who built NASA, Jim Welds, was boisterous, ebullient, and flamboyant; he would walk into a meeting with an outlandish idea, and the room would ignite. By making unreasonable requests and asking unrealistic questions, he motivated others to consider the potential of an idea. He didn't ascribe to traditional, textbook principles of management, and he didn't manage by the numbers. But people believed in his vision and his organization; after all, we did get a man on the moon.

Sony's CEO, Akio Morita, states, "Our plan is to lead the public with new products rather than ask them what kind of products they want. The public does not know what is possible, but we do." Sony introduces an average of a thousand new or updated products each year, with about 20 percent aimed at creating new markets. Many have been winners, but the Betamax VCR showed they also strike out. But Sony believes that is okay–as long as you learn!

Taco Bell, with John Martin, CEO, became aware that it was losing touch with its customers—they were not coming back. So it undertook a massive reorganization of operations and mind-set; if the food is hot, tasty, and inexpensive, all else will follow. What evolved was a team system that allowed a crew to run a restaurant without a manager. It saved money, delivered food faster, and improved employee morale. And Taco Bell discovered that a happy staff usually meant happy customers!

The myth of charismatic leaders must be understood. Though many visionary companies have had high-profile leaders like Henry Ford (the original person demanding operational excellence) or Sam Walton (who took value to the people), charismatic leadership is not necessary for success. For instance, 3M has never had a charismatic CEO.

The best leaders, charismatic or not, make it a point to develop managers and processes who respond to the environmental and community needs. In their view, the firm is not a vehicle for products or personalities; products are just a vehicle for the company's vision and image. Looked at in this light, Walt Disney's greatest creation was not *Snow White* or Disneyland; it is the Disney Company and its ability to make people a little happier, one exposure at a time.

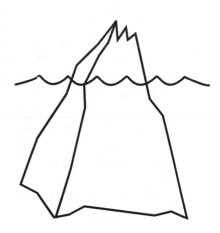

Each story shows a unique perspective, but would these leaders have had similar success stories in other corporate situations? Probably not. Many successful leaders in industry who leave their power bases fail elsewhere. Leadership is, in many ways, situational. True leadership demands that the talents of the person fit the needs of the situation.

While the style and approach of leaders may differ tremendously, there are some qualities that true leaders have in common. A positive attitude is a starting point, as well as the belief that they can make a difference regardless of the environmental stresses. Leaders have perspectives that they are able to infuse in others. They are action oriented and thus inspire others to act. Simple, concrete, and direct, they impart their philosophies in ways others can easily identify with and replicate.

- The IBM Way was based on three simple commitments, each applying to veterinary practice: respect the individual, give customers the best service, and pursue excellence.
- The Hewlett Packard Way was based on people-centered management.
- The JCPenney Way was based on the basic question "Does it square with the customer and the employee?"
- The new perspectives brought by these leaders ignited others like "People, not money or things, are an organization's greatest asset" (IBM) or "We believe our first responsibility is to the doctors, nurses, and patients, to mothers and all others who use our products and services" (Johnson & Johnson).

It is the opinion of analysts that people like Jim Welds were not born leaders, but rather, they were molded into positions of leadership through education, experience, and, most importantly, through the right opportunities. They were part of a situation that called forth leadership. During the past several years, the progressive responsiveness to community demands of individual practices as well as public corporations has been an excellent example of what people can do who are in the right spot, at the right time, with the right vision.

Veterinary practices have been slowly making the transition from detailed process management to caring administration, and by the new millennium, the community market will require we move from internal practice management to leadership within the veterinary healthcare profession *and* the community. Here are some qualities shared by community leaders in today's marketplace:

- They care about people. You can't be a leader without followers, or as Will Rogers observed, "We can't all be heroes because somebody has to sit on the curb and clap as they go by." True leaders know their power comes from people, and that is where they must make an investment.

- Leaders are willing to kill the sacred cows (they make great steaks). Imbued with a charge to change, they continually question and challenge. In doing so, they keep organizations vital, vibrant, and alive.
- They are dedicated to making their enterprises work. Full of high energy and drive, they pursue power not for its own sake but because it is the right thing for their organizations and for the community and society. Their profits flow from that philosophy.
- They become leaders by working at it. They set their career course, develop timetables, and never stop working at achieving their goals.
- They keep their lifestyle balance in perspective, balancing professional ethics, family, and net profit goals.

When incorporating these observations into veterinary healthcare delivery, there are several procedures to follow:

- Have clear goals, act on them, and share them with your employees.
- Show people how to buy into and participate in the intermediate objectives needed to reach the long-term goals; get their commitment.
- Make sure that recognition programs, including financial incentives, are targeted to the right people.
- Reward the risk takers and starve the risk avoiders. Provide loyalty to the productive staff members, not to the ones who have worked for you the longest. Merit pay must be based on past performance, not on a make no waves approach.
- Foster new leaders through delegation of authority and responsibility but do not look for carbon copies. Someone who was right a couple years ago may have no role today.

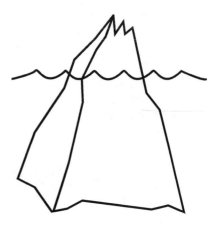

Finally, the most important task for veterinarians now is to revitalize their practice staff. Our profession has reached that mature stage in which maintenance management is not enough. Put your goals into perspective, get your staff to buy into your practice dreams, and let your people move forward with that perspective in mind.

Change Is the Norm!

Stability itself is nothing more than a more sluggish motion.
—Michel de Montaigne

To accept the nonstop change required this decade, the veterinarian must develop a new mind-set. This requires a significant transition, as the old expectations are painfully abandoned and a long, difficult adjustment must be made to an untested operational style and viable new practice.

There are times during a practice transition that neither the old systems nor the new are acceptable, and the fear of failure looms large. It isn't enough to preach about the future and share your dream. Continuous quality improvement and thriving on chaos are not rally cries when you're lost in the process of change. Changing the norm is based upon the ability to manage many small, overlapping changes one day at a time while exerting the leadership that causes the staff to follow, regardless of their fears.

The art of progress is to preserve order amid change
and to preserve change amid order.
—A. N. Whitehead

The Rumors

Continuous quality improvement is based on each person being accountable for making tomorrow better than today within his or her sphere of influence. Every new level of change in a veterinary practice will be termed nonstop by people who are having trouble with the transition. At the same time, each previous level of change, once accepted, will be called stability. Seen in this light, what the staff today call nonstop change is simply a new level of what has always existed. It isn't chaos; it's a new experience. When the staff adjust to a new method, it will represent a new stability for them.

Change is uncomfortable for about two-thirds of the U.S. population, based on known personality types. When opinions about change start taking the form of hurdles, rumor control will become essential. The rumor defuser position is that what stays constant is the expectation that every status quo is a temporary expedient until a better way to do things is discovered. Every practice improvement needs to reaffirm the unchanging values that underlie the CQI process.

Two quite opposite qualities equally bias our minds; habit and novelty.
—Jean de la Bruyere

Clarity

How often do we hear the phrase "You don't understand ..."? When staff members say this, it is a diagnostic sign that must be addressed. What is wrong with their perception of the practice? The answer is not beyond your grasp. It is a matter of pure common sense: how the staff see their activities contributing to the overall success of the practice. Their perceptions affect the mission of the practice because the staff are the implementing force.

Stability through change demands clarity about what you are trying to do. There is no reason to make an adjustment unless there is something to adjust. When change is the norm, put a premium on knowing clearly what you are trying to accomplish. What is the real mission of your practice? Liquidity? More free time? Quality healthcare services? Access to the community? An expansion plan? More clients? More patients? More staff?

Look at some commonsense missions. Ford has a mission to build vehicles that move people and things, Harvard's mission is to educate people and push the boundaries of knowledge, and your veterinary practice's mission is to provide care and treatment that cannot be given by animal owners. Each part of the practice has its own mission, from the animal caretakers in the ward to the receptionists who answer the phone. Each of their missions makes the total mission possible. If one part is not supporting the whole, it must be addressed as unjustified in the total scheme. In some cases, this means eliminating the problem agent or operation.

Far too many practices define the mission in terms of practice objectives: earning a high return on investments, practicing the best quality medicine, having a great place to work. These are important, but they are not the central, continuous thread that everyday changes are meant to preserve. It is the mission, not the objectives, that is the heartbeat of the practice. The confusion between mission and objectives has serious repercussions when change is the norm.

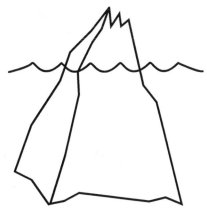

Many are stubborn in pursuit of the path they have chosen,

few in the pursuit of the goal.

—F. W. Nietzsche

The Triad

When you are ready to bring your veterinary practice into the new millennium, there are three steps to establish change as the norm: rebuild trust, unload old baggage, and sell problems rather than solutions.

Rebuild Trust

When helping a child learn to ride a bike or swim, the teacher must let go to give the child the courage to try the new skill. The teacher does not turn and walk away when letting go for the first time; he or she shadows the pupil, ready to provide the support needed to make success possible. This requires a two-sided trust based on the past experiences with the teacher and self-confidence, which for most adults is established in childhood.

Trustworthiness is encouraged by actions, not words. These directives are within your power:

1. Do what you say you will do. Don't make promises that you can't keep.

2. Listen carefully to others and tell them how you feel about what they say.

3. Understand what is important to people and work hard to protect those interests.

4. Don't build images in a dishonest manner; be truthful when explaining the whys.

5. Ask for feedback before a decision crisis; regard staff input as valuable information.

6. Don't expect more trust than you're willing to give; it must be mutual.

7. Don't equate trust with being a buddy; not all friendships are trustworthy.

8. Mistrust is a form of self-protection; most do not relinquish this safety valve easily.

9. If these eight ideas are too difficult to follow, just remind yourself of the key: Tell the truth.

Unload the Past

Memories obstruct change. You can ask for forgiveness for an old hurt, but don't expect the past not to be relived. Change attracts storms and conflicts like a magnet. Controls are removed, and old skeletons come tumbling out of the closet. While this complicates an already complicated transition, it is also an opportunity to heal old wounds that have been undermining activities.

1. The lies of the past must be acknowledged, not justified; it is the time for truth and justice.

2. Rebuilding credibility is a function of honesty, for the past and present.

3. The emergence of old scars and unresolved issues is a great gift; it represents an opportunity for organizational enhancement.

Sell Problems, Not Solutions

People let go of the past far more readily when they become dissatisfied or uncomfortable with the present. When they are convinced there is a serious problem, they look for a way to end it. Selling problems, not solutions, reinforces values and contributes to the practice's ability to embrace nonstop change:

1. When the staff understand the problem and are in the market for solutions, they don't need to be educated or informed after the fact.

2. When the boss sees the problem and the staff do not, a polarity develops, and cooperation decreases when facing the challenge.

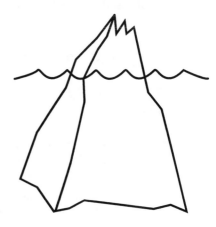

3. The more minds concentrating on the problem, the easier it is to find an integrated solution that meets the team's needs.

4. Selling problems implicates everyone in the solution, even those who abdicate.

If they choose not to be part of the solution, they cannot complain about the outcome.

When change is the norm, discovering problems is an invitation for creativity. The key to capitalizing on change lies in understanding and utilizing the cycle of challenge and response. Adversity is an opportunity to excel; inner strength is not born of prosperity but of perspiration. Innovation is the ability to respond to pressures in a unique manner that benefits more than one person. When change is the norm, the small, continuous, overlapping changes keep life exciting and frustration at bay. The end-of-chapter checklist can be used to evaluate how exciting your practice dynamics are and if you are ready to knock the socks off the competition.

The Challenge of Change

The veterinary profession is changing, for both companion animal and food animal veterinarians. The traditional male-dominated, self-sufficient, conservative practice is bending to tolerance, innovation, risk taking, integrity, credibility, networking, and specialty referrals, and that is just the beginning. Consider these provocative ideas:

- Veterinary healthcare delivery is going through a mutation. The caterpillar is becoming a butterfly or, if you are a pessimist, a moth. And whether we become butterflies or moths depends on management skills. Our fate is in our hands.
- Our age is not unlike when steamships replaced sailing ships. Captains of sailing ships didn't do very well in making the conversion. I hope that we are different.
- Old ways of living and working no longer work. It is very much like bankers in their pinstriped suits being suddenly plunked down in the tropics. All the skills they developed to survive in urban America would not only be useless but counterproductive.

Which of these analogies most approximate your current practice? There is no one practice philosophy, but we live and work in a pivotal era. Success in today's market takes many forms, but there are common threads:

- High tolerance for ambiguity and uncertainty ... the ability to make decisions and be innovative in the face of very limited information, great turbulence, and unanswered questions.
- Integrity ... the foundation of long-term relationships between organizations and their members.

- Contingency orientation ... different strokes for different folks ... an attitude and approach that always has a fallback position.
- Communication credibility ... the ability to transfer ideas with clarity, depth, interest, and excitement.
- Risk taking ... an approach in which the veterinarian's reach continually exceeds the practice's grasp.
- Delegation of authority ... diversifying the responsibilities among team members to allow the right person to meet the needs of a specific market sector ... the capability to tailor healthcare delivery to the client/patient wants and needs.

In the years ahead, our ultimate success will depend on our ability to become leaders of change. That means transforming ourselves, our organizations, and our environment. We will have to be multitalented and will have to

- Align productivity and innovation so that the organization can operate efficiently while it initiates new projects. We will pump oil from the traditional practice wells while also drilling for new ones; we will tear down while we build.
- Fuse the healing art with sound business practice. We will merge, align, and balance benevolence with bottom lines, compassion with competition, ethics with entrepreneurship. We will mold veterinary medicine into a new, diversified social enterprise.
- React to the changes that may occur within our constituencies. We will align our organizational competence with the needs and wants of our clients and eventually will come to better understand our market and colleagues' potential.
- Depend on what we see to function as efficient, lifelong learners. What we see will depend on where we choose to stand. To thrive, we will have to stand in alien places and discover new ways of looking at the world.

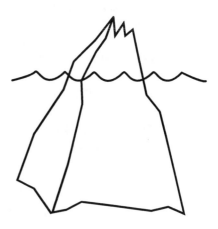

Experience may be the best teacher, but learning as a discipline will be revolutionized by the ever-shortening half-life of knowledge. Successful veterinary practices will continually be involved in a process of retooling for new discoveries.

Cataclysmic Chaos

The changes we see today are unique in history and are seen by some veterinarians as chaos. If understood, the impact may be lessened or turned into advantages.

- Traditional planning will become irrelevant. Emphasis will be on creating an adaptable organization. The five-year strategic planning programs of the past decade will succumb to the knowledge that much long-range planning involves building an unknown future on an irrelevant past.
- Small business administration and financial management will become critical practice factors. The ability to price effectively will still be limited; the net return will still be made or lost on price rather than diversity or marketing.
- Interpractice relationships will increase with technology. Shared resources at emergency clinics, referrals between practices, and long-term intersupport agreements among practices will become more commonplace.
- Independent practices will yield to corporate directorships, reducing individual liability and improving quality of life.
- With corporate umbrellas, incentive compensation programs will be developed for the new breed of entrepreneur practitioner. Motivational problems will diminish due to custom-designed benefit plans, innovation, and packages of recognition intangibles.
- The corporate overstructure will become a gardener of human potential and will learn that human resources are the only real variables in improving veterinary healthcare delivery. Nurturing will be coupled with developmental incentives to induce the changes needed.
- The traditional career paths will disappear, barriers will erode, and the trend to blame others will give way to the realization that each practice has full control of its own future if change is promoted. The chronic intraprofessional dissatisfaction with humane societies, mobile clinics, federal/state veterinary programs, and low-cost veterinary practices will be replaced by an understanding of market niche, the fact that each individual has values that cannot be met by only one practice style. Live and let live will be the philosophy, and energy will be directed toward perfecting our specific market niche for those that match our scope and style of service.

Philosophy of the Fear of Failure

That which shrinks must first expand.
That which fails must first be strong.
That which is cast down must first be raised.
That which becomes blunted must first be sharp.
That which changes shape must first be formed.
That which must be untangled was first knotted.
Before receiving, there must be giving.
This is called perception of the nature of things.

As life is a series of contrasts, so healthcare is a dichotomy. Our professional goal is to put ourselves out of business. We try to keep our patients well, but our practices depend on animals becoming sick. In curative medicine, truthful words are seldom beautiful, but beautiful words are seldom truthful. In the sciences, those who always know are not learned, but those who are learned do not always know. This is the nature of our profession.

The Fear of Change

This is a scary time for many veterinary practices. Regardless of what we have done to get where we are, it often is not enough to move forward. The old management methods no longer seem to work as well, the clients do not respond as well, and the staff—well, they are not like those we worked with before. Now is the time for leaders, for risk takers, and for innovators.

New markets have emerged, and new marketing styles are required to meet those markets. Look to the human healthcare delivery systems in your community. They now advertise, both the traditional services and the new horizontally developed wellness and ancillary services. Some have even contracted service stations to operate in their parking garages and florists to provide services in their lobbies. Many hospitals are courting additional private family practitioners to become credentialed within their systems so the hospitals can increase their inpatient bases. This evolution occurred

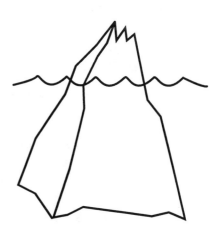

because healthcare administrators saw the future need for market niches and became the leaders and innovators their facilities needed to survive.

Veterinary medicine is not much different. It evolves in spite of the old habits and biases we carry. Veterinarians follow the leader but seldom know who is really in the lead. When I first received my Nevada license, number 278, it stated I was licensed in medicine, surgery, and dentistry, but it was 10 years later before we really discovered teeth as a potential profit center. In that same time frame I watched retail areas and boarding programs go from unethical practices, to ancillary services, and now they have become true profit centers that we need to provide to our clients.

Most families are dual income, which means someone is not available from 8:00 a.m. to 6:00 p.m. weekdays to take a pet to the veterinarian. The Saturday veterinary outpatient services have always been a madhouse, but the rest of the week was good enough that most perceived the week-end service as a favor to their clients—until this decade. Now, innovation appears to be providing evening service, longer Saturday service, and even Sunday hours. Changing hours is an acceptably safe method to differentiate services within a community. But most practices still cling to the weekday hours, even if they do not have the workload to pay the overhead. Increasing the length of the work week means there is less family and recreation time. This is not true innovation: it is a road to burnout.

In slow times, a practice may pay $100 per hour overhead to make the $46 per hour from that occasional walk-in client. From a consultant's perspective, many veterinarians live off their depreciation monies so they can have money to pay staff for doing their jobs. Practices seldom reward for innovation. Picking up the phone and bonding with clients is still a rarity in veterinary practices, regardless of the slow times. Why is this? Simply, we never had to do it before, so why start doing it now? Answer: because of competition, we must differentiate our practices from others. And when I say competition, I mean more than just professional colleagues. I mean pet stores, catalog sources, pharmacies, and feed stores that have horizontally expanded into our sacred market. How dare they!

Elements of Change

The change model is based on (1) dissatisfaction/dissent causing (2) a process to evolve that will bring about (3) new operational standards:

Change = dissatisfaction × process × model < costs.

The real problem is that all three elements need to be in equal proportions to make change occur, and in most practices, the process is an unknown. Practices may be unhappy, and some may even know where they want to be in the future, but very few have really assessed where they are, how they got there, and what systems are needed to move across the void from yesterday to tomorrow. This fear of the unknown is often translated into methods used to maintain the status quo. The status quo is safe from the risk of change, from the mistake that might prove embarrassing, or from the discovery that the old ways were detrimental to success. We all can recognize this syndrome.

A strong leader is needed to take a practice from the habits of yesterday to the model of the future. The systems needed for this transition are not the management gimmicks our profession tried in the 1980s. Rather, they are based on the principles of continuous quality improvement. The quality of a practice is determined by the client's perception of the team's pride in what it does. Each member of the veterinary healthcare delivery team needs to become accountable for making today better than yesterday. This means the practice leadership needs to promote change based on specific practice values, annual goals, and a clear philosophy. Pride cannot be felt unless expectations are exceeded, and expectations cannot be exceeded unless the standard for performance is based on competency to produce outcomes rather than adherence to traditional processes.

Leading into the Future

The ability to use innovation to achieve economic success is considered a sign of a leader. Innovation and creativity are forms of risk taking. Most veterinarians fear risk, but then so does the average person. Taking a risk in veterinary school meant using two colors of ink when taking a test. Veterinarians and technicians have traditionally been taught by rote. That is, learning meant meeting step-by-step requirements for academic fulfillment. Creativity and innovation have not been welcome in the veterinary academic community.

Harvard abandoned this process-oriented format three years ago in its medical school and has produced physicians with far better medical aptitudes, or so the clinical competency exams and intern/residency programs indicate. It expects this will also spill over into strong physician leadership in wellness medicine. Many veterinary schools have increased the preveterinary requirements, so the entering class now has more stuff to remember and apply to the curative processes being taught. This is entrenching the process, not building for the future.

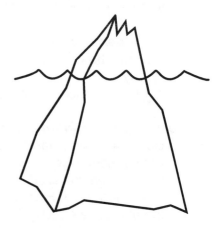

Now is the time for all technicians, receptionists, and animal caretakers to demand the opportunity to make their jobs better for the client, the patient, and themselves. Now is the time for all veterinarians to understand the characteristics and needs of the individual, to appreciate the resources within the staff, and to effectively communicate their desire to empower each person to take the risk to make the next day, week, or month better than the last. It will not be easy, and it will not be comfortable, but a full-time leader will make it happen. Leadership skills are the tenets needed to take a practice from the comfortable habits of yesterday, across the void of fear, to the prosperity of tomorrow.

Don't Procrastinate

The four killer words of progress: "I wish I could ..."

All experts on time management agree on at least one rule for getting results: Do it now! But in busy veterinary practices, tackling assignments *now* is not always as easy as it sounds. Sometimes you are not in the mood, often a critical case has distracted you from your plan, or, as in the area of management, you are overwhelmed by the size or complexity of the project. Worse, the task itself may be one that makes you uncomfortable, like performance appraisals or constructively correcting one of the staff members. Whatever the reason, or excuse, remember, "Wishing don't make it so!"

Motivation Keys

When someone on your team says, "I wish I could motivate Albert," that usually means "I wish I could get Albert to do his job better." Here are six keys to do exactly that:

Ask for performance
Describe how the job is to be done, train to that level of competency, and clearly state what you want the outcome to be. Then ask the staff member to meet those expectations within a specific time frame.

Use positive reinforcement—personalize it
Don't take acceptable work for granted; thank people for the effort. Praise them every time they improve, in process or outcome. Everyone likes to be recognized, but what motivates one may leave another cold—or even irritated. Find out what works for each team member and use the appropriate recognition style.

Build relationships

This does not mean buddy-buddy, beer-drinking, bar-hopping weekends. It means that you must understand each person on the team is an individual, with a life outside the practice. Your staff are caring human beings, and they will respond best when your actions show you respect their individuality and trust their intentions.

Understand the points of view of others

Make a habit of listening to others, at a 110 percent attention level; do not let your mind formulate replies while others are talking. Ask the opinion of teammates *before* you give directions or offer advice. If you listen first, and listen with an open mind, people are much more likely to cooperate when you decide something has to be done differently.

Model what you want

Approach your own work ethic with a sense of urgency and pride, use your time effectively, and meet the goals you set. Show staff members by your actions, not just by fancy words, that the practice philosophy really does matter—that quality is important, caring is critical, and that deadlines are real.

Refuse to accept poor performance

Motivation texts seldom address feedback for performance less than acceptable. Leaders must retrain staff members when expectations are not met. Often retraining also requires additional coaching, in which appropriate behavior is recognized and supported as it is developed. Sometimes, after retraining, reprimands are required. Leaders must clearly demonstrate that standards do matter—and that, in itself, is motivational.

It is always better to aim at excellent and hit good than to aim for good and settle for average. This is the reason that Catanzaro & Associates has, in conjunction with its continuous quality improvement programs, developed prospective performance planning methodologies for clients to replace the traditional, and uncomfortable, retrospective performance appraisals. We want to celebrate the actions and innovation of excited staff members, not support the safe, procrastinating risk avoiders.

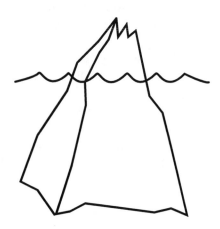

Reversing Procrastination

To procrastinate means to put off doing a task—for no good reason. Sometimes, there appear to be excellent reasons for putting off certain tasks; that is what prioritizing is all about! When this occurs, you need to look at your priority list again, regain the determination to forge ahead, and exercise the discipline to stay on track.

If you have an organized to-do list but are having difficulties acting on it, then procrastination may be the problem. Here are 10 ways to turn regret about wishes not coming true into celebration of tasks actually accomplished!

Persuade yourself

Most procrastination is the result of irrational thinking, or awfulizing. You talk yourself into putting off a task not because it is simply unpleasant but because it is awful, horrible, *unbearable!* Of course, none of these descriptions are accurate. Convince yourself that the task is worth doing, even if it is hard to get started. Look at alternative methods of beginning the job and keep in mind its positive aspects. Tell yourself, "I may not enjoy paperwork, but I can certainly understand the need for others to know what I have done; I can do it and may even feel better when it's done and others are being helped."

Discipline yourself

If you can't get started, allow yourself five minutes before starting—*only* five minutes. Set a timer and promise yourself that when the timer buzzes you will work at least five minutes on the task; when the timer buzzes, reset it and promise you will give the project your undivided attention for five minutes. Repeat this process of five-minute work intervals until doing the task is easier than resetting the timer. It is like jumping into a mountain lake in the summer; the first splash may be uncomfortable, but you soon warm to the joy of swimming.

Challenge your excuses

Argue with yourself about the reasons you use when you put something off. If you are in the habit of saying, "I work so well under pressure," argue that others around you see a harried and tired person, one that does not have the time to be creative and caring. Learn to say, "Working under pressure commits me to the *old way* and stops me from grabbing new opportunities; I need time to be innovative and responsive!" This type of positive outlook and inner debate can keep you from stalling and works for any excuse, no matter how logical it may have seemed.

Counterattack

Forcing yourself to do something uncomfortable or frightening helps to prove it wasn't that bad after all. Conducting performance appraisals for eight staff members is a task that seems to take forever, but it can be done in less than a week if, each day, an appraisal is done before work and another is completed after duty hours. A manageable goal is less threatening and gets the task accomplished. If you remain positive and forward looking, by the end of the week you will probably decide that performance planning isn't so terrible.

Develop a routine

Confirmed procrastinators usually work in a feast or famine pattern. One way to fight the tendency is to schedule frequently done tasks for regular times. Restock the commonly used items every day after lunch; this is a sluggish time when movement is far more productive than deskwork. Do filing every Friday after restocking and don't stop until everything is filed; it is your weekend that is being made worry free. Determine weekly tasks first thing Monday, 7:30 a.m. sharp, in a leader's meeting that will be adjourned *before* 8:00 a.m., regardless! You get the idea.

Remove the reward

Don't let procrastination be a pleasant experience, ever! If you usually procrastinate by socializing or doing a favorite hobby, or even just smoking a cigarette, stop it! Reserve these things as rewards *after* you finish a project. If you must procrastinate, do it in unpleasant conditions; lock yourself into catching up with filing—no cigarettes, no coffee, no visitors until you are done. When the fun goes away, so does the procrastination habit.

Write a contract

Make a written promise to yourself that states a goal, a time line, and a reward for accomplishing the goal. It can be a simple agreement: "I, Suzie, the wonder receptionist, will clear all the phone messages and run all the computer recall sheets the first thing every morning. Upon successfully completing the retrieval and routing all the messages and recalls, I will enjoy my first cup of freshly brewed flavored coffee."

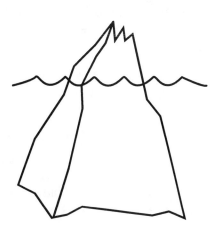

Jog your memory

Put important papers in a special folder (e.g., red) in a special place
(e.g., a vertical desk file). Tell yourself they must be done today and you
can't leave until they are completely acted upon and are out of the
folder. Put red stars by significant items on your to do list. Clear your
desk and put the most important task in the center with a Post-it note
that reads "do it!" In short, use any gimmick that keeps your attention on
the task.

Divide and conquer

Break big jobs into many small pieces and do at least one portion each
and every day. Pull the end-of-month reports off the computer and highlight the 12 critical numbers; the next day post the numbers on trend-
tracking sheets.

Post a chart

Use a chart for visible proof of your progress; it will reinforce your efforts
to stay on track. Make sure you can see it from your desk. List concurrent projects laterally if they have similar priorities. Give yourself a gold
star (or use a smiley face, a clown hat, anything that makes you smile)
for each task you accomplish in order of priority. Charting reminds you
that doing a task now—not tomorrow—makes your job easier because
work is being done in a manageable fashion.

Habits are a form of security, and procrastination is a form of security to
some. The type of music you listen to is often a result of habit. Younger
staff members may be into rap music, but the *RAP* of a practice is slightly
different although it can be as enjoyable: *r*eview the past, *a*nalyze the present, and *p*lan the future. If RAP and procrastination are discussed, steps
will generally be taken to change bad habits—by leaders first and staff
second. When priorities replace procrastination, and the rewards come,
the team will celebrate.

Team Building from the Inside

The conventional definition of management is getting work done through
people, but the real management leader develops people through work.

Most of us have played a team sport. It seems to be a requirement in the
American school system. Some people excelled, but most of us were just

good team members. We have all known poor team members, the bad sports who had to have it their way or wanted to be stars but didn't have the talent or training. We also remember the great team members, the ones who made us feel good just to share the game with them. They encouraged us while we were learning and let us star when we were ready, mentally and physically. Generally, these qualities are what we think of when we say "team player."

There are always good players, but good players are not always good team members. Remember the ball hog? Remember the pitcher who wouldn't listen to her catcher's signals, the soccer player who would pass laterally only as a panic reaction, or the volleyball player who never would set you up? That volleyball player could have been the best spiker on the net, but this didn't make you want to play another game with that person. A good team player will usually sacrifice personal glory for the good of the team. A good team leader will train others to the point they can be trusted, even in delicate situations. A good team leader can build a good team of players, and a team of good players can make the leader look good!

Inside the Veterinary Practice

Most likely, your practice has talked about team building. Some practices have accomplished it, and others are still trying to find the playing field. Most are somewhere in the middle of the process and searching for the right program. If you were selected to be a member of a healthcare delivery team, you were chosen for a reason, so teamwork must be an expectation of the practice. The primary reason that a practice team doesn't come together is that no one has shared the rules for winning. We know how wide the football field is and how points are scored. We know where the three-point line is on the basketball court and what happens if we commit a foul. Heck, most of us even know the rules for winning a billiard game (we saw the movie *The Hustler*).

In the veterinary practice, achieving a goal is how the practice scores, and the technical manual, job descriptions, and employee manual are the rule books for the game. The ability of a veterinary practice to discuss these elements in a clear and concise manner is a critical element of team building. In Catanzaro & Associates, we call it "train to trust." If a practice leader or manager does not trust someone, the training has been deficient, not the person. How the practice philosophy, core values, and operational principles (performance standards) are shared sets the tone for team play. In many practices, job descriptions have been replaced by the authority to solve problems within established guidelines instead of by the rule book. You can't win unless you know how to score points using the team's, or practice's, playing capabilities.

A Good Team Player

If you are a good team player, if you really are trying to build a team to deliver veterinary healthcare to patients that need your skills, then you will have these attributes:

1. You will be committed at the beginning and play hard all the time. You will not sit out on a play and then say, "I told you so." You will expose your thoughts and feelings for the team to view and evaluate. This is open feedback. You may disagree, but you won't ever try to make someone else wrong. It takes courage to be this type of team player.

2. If you don't know the practice goal or objective, you will find a way to define it. You will share this knowledge with others on the team. Because you care, you will question the unknown.

3. You will help determine how to accomplish the practice goals and objectives. You will seek input from others and understand that their input is important to practice improvement; practice enhancement equals team success. You will believe that your contribution is equally important to the practice and to the team's success.

4. You will see the good intentions of other team members. You will praise the good they have attempted to do before discussing how to do a job better next time. You will sacrifice your independence for team intradependence, and you will respect the skill and expertise of others. You will ensure you understand the good reasons for another's ideas *before* you offer contrary opinions.

5. Decision making is a group effort that requires a volunteer on some occasions. A veterinary extender (proactive staff member) is someone who sees a need and finds a way to fulfill it without creating extra workload for the doctor or other staff members.

6. You will share the success; you won't backpedal in the light of failure. You will share credit for the good ideas that have worked. A good team shares the glory, but a great team celebrates the success of oth-

ers. In the event of adversity, you will seek information and improve the system to prevent recurrence.

Personal Roles on the Team

You may become a team star, but even the best stars never forget how they became known. At the end of his last season Joe Montana said that he was good *only* because of the other 10 team members on the field. A pass can't be caught by the thrower, a handoff requires someone else to run, and even a quarterback sneak takes a lot of blocking by the line. Never forget that it is the team score that is entered into the record book, that the team wins the trophy, and that every member of the team gets a Super Bowl ring. In veterinary practice, a team scores when a client comes back or when the client refers a friend to the practice. The *front door must swing* for a score to occur! No one cares how much you know until they know how much you care. Caring brings clients back.

In veterinary healthcare, it is the individual members of the team who influence the client's perception of the quality of care, who deliver concerned care to the pet, and who make the practice a pleasure to be at for staff, clients, and veterinarians. It isn't easy to be a great team player. Continuous quality improvement (CQI) requires that you take pride in the daily routine and your contribution to practice excellence. Most all clients equate an individual's staff member's pride with quality.

The basic concept of CQI is that you own your team contributions and that you will make tomorrow a little better than today for yourself, the patient-client pair, and the practice. You will seldom be noticed for what you deserve, but the team will be seen as very effective. A good team member will know that he or she has contributed to this image and will find it is a pleasure to go to work!

Beyond Sports

An athlete can go to the dressing room to recuperate after a hard-played four-hour game. It is not that way in a veterinary practice. You are in the center of the action for hours on end, until patient demand and client needs wane.

In team sports, the conditioning is both physical and mental, within the demands of the sport. The limitations placed on the opponents are well-defined, so the efforts of the team are directed toward looking for

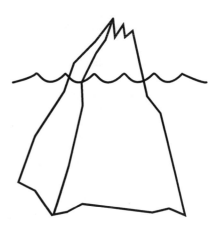

weaknesses. In veterinary medicine, diseases and bodily injury have no limitations. Mutations occur as well as accidents. Problems are the rule, not the exception. There is no time-out or instant replay. The conditioning is mental and physical. The unexpected is the usual.

The veterinarian is the quarterback, the coach, the manager, and, during many night emergencies, often the rest of the team. When the staff members assume the role of paraprofessional veterinary extenders, they commit to a life of dynamic change, to excitement based on the unknown and unpredictable, to a set of rules that are changed by every client encounter and every patient healthcare situation. The requirement to think for yourself is a necessity in a healthcare emergency. A practice leader understands this and offers continual in-service training so every member of the team can be trusted to respond to the crisis of the moment with competency and caring.

There is a team synergy in veterinary healthcare delivery, and it makes the support of patient needs come naturally. The empathy felt toward team members in times of stress is usually translated into physical as well as moral support. The stressed client is not a spectator but rather someone who needs the team's care and concern. A great team player learns to see healthcare services through the eyes of the client. When the client perceives a higher practice quality because of this team member's efforts, then a successful team play is achieved.

The veterinary practice system demands that the professional and paraprofessional staff make a greater commitment based on trust and caring, skill and competency, sacrifice and personal tenacity. This does not require a playbook, an umpire, or a sideline coach. It requires a specialized healthcare delivery team that is able to establish a set of common values that guide members' decisions and action.

The following is the summary from *Managing from the Heart,* by Bracey, Rosenblum, Sanford, and Trueblood.

Hear and understand me.

Even if you disagree, please don't make me wrong.

Acknowledge the greatness within me.

Remember to look for my caring intentions.

Tell me the truth with compassion.

Make it your challenge to meet these practice, staff, and client needs.

Survival-Based Innovation

Life is lived forward but understood backward.
—Søren Kierkegaard

Veterinarians are like engineers—they love numbers. Numbers make them feel secure. The engineer has his stress test, and the veterinarian has the client transaction. As practices grow, they tend to lose sight of what built their practice: client-centered service, quality healthcare, and a caring approach to staff and client needs. Instead, they start to manage by numbers. Practice owners begin to worry more about the efficiencies of the staff and less about the needs of the community. Good practice leaders must maintain their intuitive feel for client attitudes, community needs, and market trends. They should look at the numbers, but they should not be ruled by them.

Innovation Is Disruptive

As a practice grows, veterinarians seek operating efficiency in order to drive expenses lower. The innovation originally targeted at the front door (gaining new clients) is often retargeted to internal operations. The practice seeks to develop protocols to produce repetitive, replicable, and reliable performance by the staff. This drive to standardize often makes the staff miss the opportunities to expand.

The protocol mind-set inhibits innovation because the organization processes that foster efficiency are often diametrically opposed to those that foster innovation and creativity. Efficiency calls for coordination, streamlining, and eliminating slack and waste wherever feasible. Innovation, on the other hand, is often messy and wasteful and creates a climate of experimentation, false starts, and trial and error. It requires ample resources to thrive. In human healthcare, a 20 percent success rate for innovation in client service is considered high.

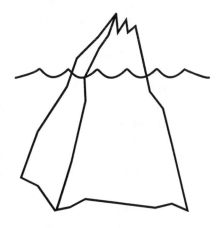

Veterinarians usually want projections before they start a new program, yet new and emerging markets often defy projections. Client surveys may not reveal a sufficient number of interested clients to justify the new program. But then, the interested clients may not yet be coming to the practice because the program doesn't exist. For instance, in 1976 very few people considered themselves in need of a personal computer. And in the early 1980s, IBM was focusing so hard on the PC that it missed the need for laptop computers and has had to play catch up ever since.

Creativity is often the key to new markets. The American Animal Hospital Association (AAHA) discovered a market for dental care in the 1980s, offered specialized courses, and started a trend toward dental hygiene never seen before in our profession. Animals had teeth when I graduated, heck, even before I graduated. But it took the AAHA's creativity to make treatment of them an acceptable market. Markets can be created. Catanzaro & Associates coaches a practice in Duluth that wanted to do more ophthalmology, but it did not offer the care because of the cost. We convinced the practice that the clients had the right to say no, and many did. But many have said yes. The practice of ophthalmology is now a weekly occurrence rather than a monthly rarity. A practice in Michigan offered a pet fat farm program after the Christmas holidays; it included two weeks inpatient, with laboratory monitoring twice a week and a refeeding program to get the pet onto a new, healthier diet. A significant segment of the clients considered this innovative service needed care since they couldn't face "starving" their pets.

Substantiation of market need cannot always be reduced to a science. The preceding two programs would not have worked for a couponing practice that lives on low prices and volume. When leaders desire a team that capitalizes on opportunities, adapts to change, and promotes innovation, they must stop trying to predict the unpredictable.

Conservative practices play the game not to lose, versus the innovative practice that continually plays to win. Nike plays with its product line continuously, regardless of the success of the existing products. An entire range of sport shoes has been developed from the original sneaker era. The capacity to innovate is critical to outperforming others in a dynamic environment. It is imperative for every veterinary practice to understand the six basic alternatives available for promoting innovation.

Innovation based on core technologies

New products are exploited, like dental points, dental bases, electric power drills, as well as actual services, like root canals and teeth polishing. The dry chemistry machines have brought STAT laboratory capabilities back into the private practice setting. 3M's innovation in adhesives has resulted in surgical glues, medical tapes, and incise drapes.

Innovation based on a unique remix of common operating elements

Client-centered practices believe that what is done is less the source of innovation than the manner in which it is done. Using telephone follow-ups and reminders has increased the liquidity of many practices simply because the clients perceived the calls as caring. Hill's has tried to put a nutrition center in every practice, but very few practices have assigned a nutritional counselor to every overweight patient. The ones that have produce greater liquidity because technicians can be cost-effective in this environment while the veterinarian's time is cost-prohibitive. Using a topic-specific, red-bordered health alert (instead of a newsletter), then following it with a call to action practice promotion (specialty clinic) three weeks later, delivers routine services in a unique manner. Even using a progressive and repetitive client relations training program for receptionists is a unique remix in some communities.

Innovation that satisfies unmet client needs

Clients' needs may only be their wants: a feline-exclusive practice, where dogs cannot disturb cats, an exclusive species approach to facility design, the first avian practice promoted in the community, a "traveling with your pet" promotion to get all dogs on heartworm preventative a month before they depart, or an evening (4:00 to 8:00 p.m.) satellite vaccination clinic in a bedroom community subdivision where harried commuters live.

Innovation created from pure imagination

Disney studios coined the term "imagineering" to describe its philosophy for market interactions. Innovation created from pure imagination may be something like the pet fat farm program or something as uncommon as a unique client-centered, full color hospital brochure. Computer software is in this niche, mainly because its search-and-sort and query capabilities access relationships never seen before. To determine specific doctor continuing education (CE) needs before a geriatric pet promotion program is launched, some practices offer dogs older than seven years ECGs followed up with thoracic X rays.

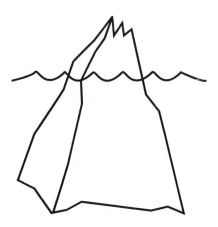

Innovation based on scientific research

In the early days of our profession, innovation based on scientific research was often the wonder drug. But the cost-effectiveness of human healthcare technological systems has made orthopedics, ultrasound, and endoscopy practical for veterinary medicine. Also, insulin is now genetically engineered, and technological advances have made embryo transplants commonplace in food animals.

Innovation based on functional excellence

Board-certified specialists have left the university setting and are flourishing in the private practice, metroplex environment. There are free-standing ophthalmology-exclusive practices now—what specialty will be next? Imaging centers have started to proliferate in human medicine. Are we next? In the average practice, value-added services include one-stop shopping, identification tattooed on pets under anesthesia for dental work or a spay, and practice technicians offering behavior management assistance utilizing the new canine head collar.

The Competitive Advantage

It is imperative that innovation be channeled into a competitive advantage. When a unique idea is implemented, the clients must be told. I have seen a practice that offers home veterinary care for shut-ins but lists the service under a separate name. It is never associated with the parent facility. I have seen other practices staff to support morning drop-off of day care patients but not tell clients about it in their hospital brochures because they acquired too much inpatient business when they did. It does a practice very little good to offer innovative services without the client's knowledge.

Clients must perceive the innovation as unique. It must set the practice apart from others in the community. This is why the low-cost vaccination and spay clinics benefit those who first introduce the services in a community. Clients may flock to clinics offering sale prices, but the clinics are the first to close in tight economic times, since there is no client loyalty and other discounts attracted the clients elsewhere.

Boarding and resale pet supplies at veterinary hospitals were innovative, became commonplace, and then were considered nonprofessional in the 1970s. When the Federal Trade Commission had a short discussion with the national veterinary associations in the mid-1980s, image-based ethics were put into abeyance, and now innovative practices have again built resale outlets and boarding facilities as one-stop shopping conveniences. Maintaining a competitive advantage is difficult, since the unique becomes common when copied by others. To sustain it, practices must combine creativity, innovation, and human resource management skills.

Maximizing the yield of innovation requires management. For instance, one full-time animal caretaker can support 33 animals in an eight-hour day, so boarding facilities must be built and managed to ensure this level of occupancy so that the employee is effectively utilized. Does this mean building a megafacility and marketing toward a 60 percent occupancy or does it mean a staff of part-time college kids who can have their hours adjusted to meet the demand? Does it mean changing the ratio of cat condos with windows to sterile stainless steel cages or does it mean increasing the eight-foot run capacity of the facility to meet the large dog demands? Or is it another combination of alternatives not yet evaluated? These questions are community and practice specific.

Market share is seldom stolen from a practice. It is just let go by not meeting the wants and needs of the clients. Clients who bond to a practice are forgiving but not dumb. The veterinary client of today is well educated. Televisions provide information on pet wellness on a regular basis. The average pet owner is blasted with marketing information multiple times a day. Current research suggests at least 75 percent of pet owners consider their pets members of the family and about a third of these give their companion animals people status. The client-centered practice understands this, offers the best and most unique services available, and lets the client decide whether or not they are needed.

The pace of change has increased in every aspect of veterinary healthcare, from staff capabilities to graduate skills to client education levels. Chemotherapeutics and equipment have changed, competitors have increased, and distribution channels have proliferated. Practices that do not, will not, or cannot innovatively adapt to these changes will pay the price. Those practices that keep the blinders on are easy to spot. Their net has decreased for two to three years. The gross may be have increased, but it is the net that pays for new equipment, debt retirement, and a better quality of life. Innovation that promotes a distinctive competitive advantage promotes a distinctive liquidity for the veterinary practice.

Nonstop Change—A Manager's Checklist

Yes No

___ ___ Have I accepted the fact that nonstop change is unavoidable in veterinary practice today?

___ ___ Have I quit making excuses for the past?

___ ___ Do I have a design for where the practice is going so my staff can connect the dots to reach success?

___ ___ Am I orchestrating my transition management tactics effectively, moving from change-triggered chaos to defined endings and new beginnings?

___ ___ Am I careful not to introduce operational definitions into the practice's core values?

___ ___ Am I firmly focused on the present needs and not staking too much on the future?

___ ___ Have we made life cycle projections of existing programs to identify and start developing replacement programs and systems?

___ ___ In team discussions are we addressing the worst case scenarios for forecasted as well as current actions?

___ ___ Do I perceive the staff moving from occasional change to change the norm thinking?

___ ___ Is the status quo accepted as a temporary resting place in the practice's change process?

___ ___ Has the team agreed (and does it understand) that change is the best way to ensure the continuity of the practice?

___ ___ Have I made the practice mission clear enough to be differentiated from the objectives of the practice?

___ ___ Do I have deep feelings about the mission, rather than just paying lip service to it?

___ ___ Am I working regularly to sell the practice problems to the staff in an honest and truthful manner?

___ ___ Did I take action today to reinforce that change is the norm of this practice?

Application Exercise

As stated in the Introduction, mind mapping is an excellent technique not only for generating ideas but also for developing intuitive capabilities. Use the iceberg ideas you have added on the odd-numbered pages and the concepts you have drawn from this chapter to expand the following mind map.

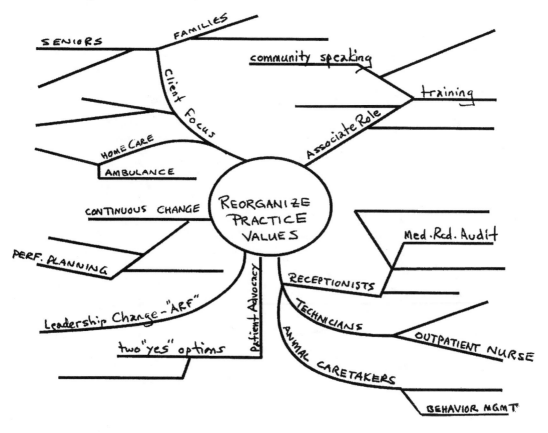

The Right Person for the Right Job

Staff members are the gems of a practice, cherish them!
—Dr. T. E. Cat

Chapter One offers some ideas for redesigning the organization of veterinary practices—ways to look at old habits to see something new. The same must be done for the people portion of the practice. The old trend was to replace ineffective staff while the new trend is to train and retain the staff as valuable assets of the practice. This requires *leadership!*

Listening—listening to others attentively, with an open mind

Ethics—doing the right things, for the right reasons, at the right time

Ambition—goals, imagination, and vision, backed by ability

Desire—enthusiasm, drive, and determination make the practice better

Example—role models, ideals, honesty, common sense, and hard work

Respect—respect for others, self, clients, patients, and life

Self-esteem—poise and belief in self, nothing to prove to others

Heart—empathy, nurturing, and encouragement

Innovation—energy and ability to see things in a new way

Patience—slow to criticize, quick to praise

Job Redesign

Work is for man and not man for work.
—Pope John Paul II

The use of job descriptions has become popular in veterinary medicine to protect the hiring process as well as to establish minimum expectations. Other healthcare professions used these in the early 1980s, then went on to establish corporate or hospital values in the late 1980s. Now the same group of healthcare administrators is looking at job redesign as a method to increase recognition and productivity.

Job redesign refers to the process of determining what tasks and work processes will comprise a given job or group of interrelated jobs. It typically involves either job enrichment or job enlargement. Under both job enrichment and job enlargement, paraprofessionals are continually developed to a higher level of performance. *Job enlargement* is nothing new; it involves increasing the number of operations that an individual performs in a given job cycle. The jobs are roughly at the same skill level, as discussed by Herzberg in the *Harvard Business Review* as long ago as 1968. *Job enrichment* requires a healthcare leader, not just a manager. When a job is enriched, the individual assumes higher-level functions and responsibilities not previously delegated to him or her.

Originally, Hackman and Oldham, authors of *Work Redesign,* extended the understanding of job enrichment with the Job Diagnostic Survey questionnaire, which measured perceptions of the degree to which jobs were enriched. The five dimensions of a job that are most applicable to enrichment for the paraprofessional healthcare worker usually involve nonroutine tasks:

1. Skill variety—the degree to which a job requires a variety of different skills.

2. Task identity—the degree to which a job requires completion of a whole or identifiable piece of work.

3. Task significance—the degree to which a job has a substantial impact on the lives of other people.

4. Autonomy—the degree to which a job provides substantial freedom, independence, and discretion.

5. Feedback—the degree to which carrying out the activities required by

the job results in the individual obtaining direct and clear information about the effectiveness of his or her performance.

Job Productivity and Job Redesign

Job enlargement is more common than job enrichment in veterinary practices. If someone does well, give that person more to do. There has not been much evidence that job enlargement increases employee productivity, although some healthcare workers have said it reduces the monotony of duties. The increase in job variety is helpful in improving job satisfaction and attendance, but the main problem remains: the basic nature of the job does not change.

Job enrichment increases the employee's authority, responsibility, and autonomy. Consequently, job enrichment provides greater intrinsic rewards to employees. An early study done at the American Telephone and Telegraph Company (AT&T) indicated that job enrichment significantly increased productivity and job satisfaction while reducing turnover. However, a more recent review by Kopelman in *National Productivity Review* indicates that job enrichment has a greater influence on the quality of performance than the quantity of performance. Job enrichment also appears to lower absenteeism and turnover as well as improve job satisfaction.

A word of warning about the Hawthorne Effect. The Hawthorne Effect was the discovery that any group showed improvement when studied by an outside agency, regardless of system changes. Improvement in productivity and job satisfaction occurred just because the workforce felt someone cared. In some cases, changes in the work layout, technology, training, compensation, or the role of the supervisor under observation accompanied the job redesign being studied and influenced the final observations, but this does not really matter, as long as the proper measurements were established to recognize improvements as they were made.

Parameters of Job Redesign

Any approach to job redesign is more likely to be effective if it considers the organizational conditions (the hospital facility and philosophy) in which the task is performed as well as the nature of the healthcare delivery team involved. In considering the feasibility of job redesign within any veterinary practice, certain preexisting conditions must be evaluated:

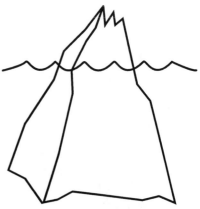

✓existing contract limitations
✓technology constraints
✓budget flexibility
✓internal control and operational audit procedures
✓technical skill of paraprofessional team members
✓leadership techniques of the hospital management team

Supervisor and middle management resistance is the rule not the ex-ception when attempting job redesign. To give someone authority and ac-countability in solving problems as they arise, the same accountability and authority must be taken away from middle management. In fact, in human healthcare, the concept of "divisions" within the hospital organization has almost disappeared; it was a layer of management not required when paraprofessional teams became empowered to solve problems at the worker level. As such, retraining and possibly redirecting the supervisors is critical to making any job redesign effort successful; in some cases, other inducements may be required, so remain flexible.

The concept of problem solving at the worker level gave rise to the prin-ciples of continuous quality improvement (CQI) in the 1990s. CQI is sim-ply establishing a hospital environment that encourages every healthcare delivery team member to have pride in personal performance; the quality of the performance is determined by the receiver of that effort. The suc-cess of job redesign, or even CQI, is based on establishing certain hospi-tal environmental conditions:

■ Management emphasizes job enrichment over job enlargement, even though the latter is the easier method of job assignment.
■ Organizational factors, such as habits, traditions, and technology, are not cause for constraints; rather, they are opportunities to excel.
■ Middle management and other traditionalists are provided with ap-propriate inducements to support job redesign.
■ Employee compensation as well as recognition is increased along with skills and responsibilities.
■ Redesign is a voluntary process targeted to individuals with a high need for growth and achievement.

Impact of Job Redesign

There have always been wide variations in compensation levels and in the ways that salary levels are determined. There should not be a pursuit of national averages but, rather, a sensible plan based on productivity, per-formance, and recognition factors. Each veterinary practice must establish a baseline and a progression plan based on its own historical liquidity. In human healthcare, the base salary was not adjusted in the majority of the job redesign cases; in the other cases the base salaries were adjusted in relatively small increments (typically less than 8 percent).

The most significant response by paraprofessionals involved in job redesign was that the job was made more interesting. From the management viewpoint, benefits included cost containment, efficiency improvements, enhanced flexibility of staffing, greater availability of service, easier employee recruitment, and higher morale. Cost containment was most significant when the job redesign combined enlargement and enrichment with no difference in base pay. Most respondents, paraprofessionals, and management perceived a positive impact on the quality of care; the perceived impact was greater at hospitals that implemented a pay differential for additional skills and authority.

Veterinary medicine will never pay competitive salaries unless the quality of life and personal recognition intangibles become components in the compensation formula. Job redesign and job enrichment will be critical to that process.

Hiring Winners

In veterinary practice, we do not hire people to do jobs, we hire them to

solve problems. The sooner the practice leader understands this,

the sooner practice growth begins.

—Dr. T. E. Cat

There are four steps in the staff procurement process: attraction, selection, retention, and attrition. Practices attract potential staff members in different ways, but the applicants come due to a certain set of community and practice values that are perceived in the practices. Selection is easier when the appropriate applicants are attracted. Once applicants are hired, retention and attrition must be considered if the new members are to be developed into practice winners.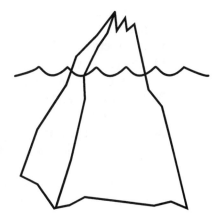

Given the high costs of finding and training new employees, you can't afford a hiring mistake. The challenge in today's veterinary practice is to find capable and qualified candidates who are going to stick with the practice. On some occasions we only offer a salary that lures the substandard applicant, but that is because we do not think of the cost involved in bringing him or her up to the level of a highly qualified applicant. We want to hire team members who extend our caring professional services, and a well-planned search and decision-making system can help ferret out winners.

Personnel agencies and help-wanted pages should be last resorts. The screening process is time-consuming, and good candidates may be missed due to poorly written resumes. Instead, use the appropriate professional society or trusted colleagues for direct referrals; the advantage of this approach is that members of professional organizations are likely to be committed. Try to find the great restaurant hostess when filling a receptionist position or seek assistance from a nurse's aide vocational school for a technician assistant candidate; this approach puts you in control of candidate selection. Movers and shakers will offer their business cards to the great restaurant hostess for "when the hostess gets tired of the food business." The search for excellent leads is a never-ending process, but the office application file for a receptionist position would be adequate if we took time to make those unsolicited inquiries to people we were impressed by.

The Job Model

Hire for personal strengths and attitude; train for skills!
—Catanzaro & Associates

Steer away from job descriptions, those laundry lists of tasks, except as a starting point. They seldom reflect the real practice philosophy. Develop job models that characterize the nature of the work. They should include

- Achievable results (what you would like to see the person accomplish)
- Obstacles (realistic problems expected in the practice operation)
- The job environment (physical space, reporting relationships, and the pace of the practice)
- An updated summary of activities from the people who already do the functions
- The management, or work style, required (ability to handle pressure, stress, and delegated authority)

When filling an existing position, review the job model before the job is advertised to see if it needs to be rewritten.

- Ensure that it is complete and will be clear and concise for the reader.
- Ask staff members to write the common traits needed to be effective within the position.
- Make sure the achievable results include objectives for the coming year.
- Review the practice philosophy and mission statement as well as the quarterly goals and objectives.

Before you interview the candidates, give them the job model, a clinic brochure, and the employee handbook (practice policy letters).

Another tip: when you place the ad, give a false name so that when Ms. Sherman is requested you will be alerted that an applicant is calling.

The Phone Interview

Start the hiring process with a phone interview that incorporates knock-out questions. The phone interview can be ceased at any time and allows evaluation of phone technique and communication skills. Have the resumes hand delivered, without an interview time, so you can get a first impression before the actual interview day. Referring to resumes before or after the phone interview is a personal preference but may depend on the position being filled, so be flexible. Interviewing prospective employees by phone requires techniques different from those used in person. But it can be much more efficient than face-to-face meetings, particularly when you have a long list of candidates to screen or when you are selecting a new receptionist who will be your phone representative. Here is how to make telephone interviews work:

List knockout questions

Base questions on the qualities or skills you decided the job requires. The knockout questions may be about commitment to emergency hours, team cooperation, experience, or simply values. For example: "How much advance notice would you need to work after 5:00 p.m.?" If the candidate does not respond positively to this question, you can end the interview—an option you can't exercise gracefully in a face-to-face situation. There is no reason to waste your time—or the applicant's.

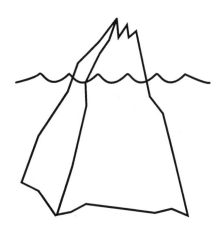

Phrase questions neutrally

Don't give away answers you want to hear. Instead of asking, "Do you work well on your own?" ask, "Is it your style to work on your own or with a team?" Neutral questions really work better in phone interviews than face-to-face since there are no visual cues possible. The answers received will be more candid and will give you a better sense of compatibility.

Design a ratings format

You are more likely to confuse candidates and their qualifications if you interview by phone because you have no visual memory jogs. That is why a written score is critical: one to five, pluses or minuses, or even letter grades, whatever works for you. Please note that although yes and no questions are easier to score they tend to mask true feelings. Mix the questions to properly assess the candidates. Make your screening selection based on the highest score.

Keep calls to applicants confidential

If you call people where they work, ask whether or not they are free to talk candidly. If not, offer to call them at home. If you must leave a message, just leave your name and number, not the practice name.

Be direct

Explain that you are calling to get more information before making the decision about whom to interview at your office. If you get a negative response to a knockout question that is critical, say that a positive answer was imperative to be considered and thank the applicant for his or her time. If candidates meet the essential requirements and possess the desirable qualities, simply state that you will assess the information and will get back to them within a particular period of time. This is also the time to ask them if they have any questions and to see if they wish to decline further interviewing.

It is important to get back to everyone you talked to during the screening process. Phone the people you want to see; write letters to those you eliminate as candidates. An employer who doesn't do this jeopardizes future relationships with job candidates as well as the practice's reputation within the community.

The Next Step in Hiring Winners

After the phone-screening procedure, candidates asked to interview at the practice should be provided the job model. Allow them adequate time to read it and also allow them to ask questions about it. The conversation that follows should be a direct effort to match the candidate with the position. Both of you should be able to tell very quickly whether or not there is a basis for further discussion.

It would be smart to schedule an interview at 7:00 on a Monday morning if you are worried about substance abusers. Be ready to watch body language at this hour. Each interview increases the chances of uncovering problems. Applicants are on their best behavior, making early detection of these problems difficult. If someone is late for an interview, that person will be late to work. I would not hire the applicant unless Mother Nature shut down the city.

One innovative approach to interviewing job applicants is to use a screening team: a receptionist, a technician, plus one other, such as an employed veterinarian, client, or bookkeeper, depending on the position to be filled. This team should ask questions that will elicit information about the candidate's experience and skills. Finding out about these areas is a straightforward exercise when the team makes a list of questions based on the job model, resumes, and job knowledge (and be sure to ask the same set of questions of every candidate, even if you like a particular person). In fact, if the receptionist and technician are to be the primary trainers, make them the primary hiring decision makers.

Interview Questions

The questions are the interview cornerstone and the responses the indicators that should be heard before a decision is made. It is the responsibility of the interviewer to get the person to reveal inner values. I have attached Appendix C, which includes a list of common interview questions; please feel free to steal any ideas to develop an interview script for your practice. When formulating the interview questions, there are a few basic parameters to follow:

1. As in the phone interview, avoid questions that can be ended with yes or no answers; ask questions that will reveal the thought process. For instance, "Do you like your current job?" could be rephrased as "What do you like about your current job?" Determining candidates' knowledge level is tricky. "What if" scenarios about working situations can help uncover how much they know about their field and what steps they would take or methods they would ap-

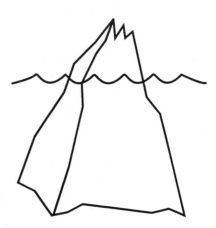

ply to solve a problem. Throughout the interview, listen for "how" and "why" explanations and examples of real accomplishments.

2. Use neutral ground to establish basic values, such as questions about the applicants' best job following high school.

3. Comparison or contrast techniques result in insights not usually provided in an interview. Ask candidates to compare or contrast two previous workplaces based on the predominant management style; you will be surprised what they perceive as management style as well as the replies themselves. Elicit evaluations of others, such as the traits of the best supervisor they ever had, the hardest person they ever trained, or the characteristics of the role model that influenced them the most in their lives.

4. Ask them to evaluate themselves from the perspectives of previous bosses, peer groups, or families. Another use of self-evaluation is to ask them to give examples of their best traits—are they conservative, creative, people persons?

5. Become blunt; ask them what they need the most help to learn, what aggravates them in the workplace, or what kinds of people are turnoffs to them.

6. Don't be afraid of hypothetical questions; they often reveal more about the applicant than other type of question does. For example, "What would you do if a person came running through the door carrying a dog that was just hit by a car? It is bleeding all over the reception room floor, and the person states that he is not the owner but it happened right in front of the hospital so he brought the dog to you." Would you expect applicants to address the healthcare needs before the economic needs, or do you want them to route the person and dog into the exam room to move the panic and trauma out of the reception area? Great question, tough answer. If you allow the HBC dog into an exam room, medical courts in most states would rule that you accepted the case and were responsible for treatment to the best of your medical ability. You have to have a clearly defined practice philosophy before you ask a question like this.

7. When using penetrating questions (why, what, how, who), learn to use silence as an interview technique; ask the leading question and then be quiet. The first person to speak loses. Learn to repeat the key words of candidates, then be silent to get them to expand upon their thoughts.

Some of the once traditional questions are not allowed to be asked by federal law: those concerning marital status, dependent children, health status, age, and nonwork social preferences—questions that may be based on bias or prejudice. Most American organizations, including schools, can't even release information favorable to the candidate, due to "equal disclosure."

The Evaluation

By definition, the employment interview is a two-way discussion, with both people giving and getting information. The information is exchanged to determine compatibility between qualifications and needs. Relevant information must take precedence over feel good exchanges between the players. The universal fact in modern interview theory is that *past performance and behavior are the most reliable factors for predicting future performance and behavior.*

While questions will vary depending on the position being filled, the score sheet for any interview should have five parts:

✓education (the ability to study and learn from text)
✓knowledge (the ability to apply theory to workplace and life)
✓experience (learning from life encounters)
✓skills (ability to perform specific tasks effectively)
✓personal attitude (required for other factors to be beneficial)

Within each of the five areas, select the questions that will most likely reveal the key characteristics. Predetermine the minimum requirements needed for someone to join the team.

New staff members are entering a practice family. It is uncomfortable for all concerned. Evaluation of the replies must include an assessment of values of the existing staff: Will the new candidate fit into the team? Have you stated the practice values as they exist, not as you wish they were? Did you ask the candidate how he or she would help solve a value issue within the practice?

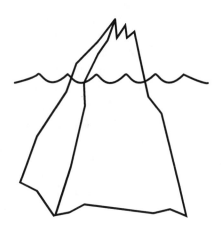

Unquestionably, a winning attitude is needed in today's veterinary practice, so phrase some questions specifically to determine if the candidate has a positive or negative attitude. Do not confuse confidence with a positive attitude; some of the most negative people are confident.

A sample interview guide for hiring receptionists appears in Appendix C. It is scored by + and – marks and can be used by everyone on the interview team. The factors included in the sample form allow interviewers to evaluate a potential team member from many perspectives. The questions and the "what to listen for" guidelines need to be tailored to the specific practice and the specific responsibilities that the new employee will assume. The characteristics of a great accounts receivable specialist will not match the traits needed by a telemarketing representative. In fact, we should hire for attitude first, then for the specifics of the position at hand; a person with the proper attitude will be able to do the job with adequate training on the practice's part.

After the interview, each team member should assign a quantitative value of how he or she feels the person measures up to the job model. The same evaluation must be used for every candidate. If the team is composed of a front room person, a back room person, and a business office person, the harmony of their evaluations will help identify the top candidates. This method will also test the objectivity of each of the team members, so the discussion after completing the rating of each applicant will help confirm impressions or point up inconsistent conclusions that need re-evaluation.

Check references with the understanding that court actions and litigations have made them virtually worthless. Most smart organizations will not give out honest information, so be ready to uncover information with questions such as "Is this person eligible for rehire?" I don't know of any animal facilities that have an internal policy against rehire, so if the person is not eligible, it is usually safe to assume that person left under unfavorable circumstances.

The Final Step in Hiring Winners

The Orientation

Most every practice has a *dis*orientation program—a half-day session to get the feel of the facility—followed by the on-the-job-training ordeal. This lightweight approach to training employees causes confusion, insecurity, and low productivity. IBM has decided that 16 weeks are required for an orientation. Trial-and-error costs money and occasionally costs clients. The American Animal Hospital Association has an exceptional set of receptionist training tapes with workbooks, but even they need to be adapted to the practice's philosophy and comfort zone.

Do not let your new employees bump into walls and injure their self-image. I recommend a 30-day orientation, then 30 days of on-the-job training, then a 30-day fire-free attempt to operate within the practice. This 90-

day probationary period can be called a "temporary hire" or "trial" period. It needs to be a supervised development time when all the basics can be covered and the person's strengths evaluated before final hiring occurs.

For example, the receptionist or technician hiring team can guide the candidate in an orientation period at a lower wage (because this is a non-productive time when the employee gains experience working at the practice), and then the team can meet with Doc to set the new wage when the person is ready to go solo for the remainder of the 90-day introductory hiring period. At the end of the 90-day period (with no benefits), the boss can again meet with the key team members to determine the real status of the candidate's capabilities, competencies, and team fit. If there isn't a team fit, do not hire for skills!

The Final Selection

The boss is best suited to making the final selection and determining the salary. There may be only one or two applicants selected for the hospital director to interview. During the orientation period, the hospital director must establish performance standards and empower the receptionist and technician trainers in the eyes of the candidate. The probation period must be clearly defined and the method(s) of performance appraisal explained before the job is offered. Expectations must be crystal clear to the prospective employee. In fact, one closing interview statement that stands out in my memory is "If you don't plan to sweat, don't take this job."

The Exit Interview

When an employee leaves your practice, try to assess why. Sometimes an exit interview is possible and will shed some light onto the situation. The reason most employees leave their jobs prematurely is that their expectations are different from their employers'. If that is applicable to your practice, it is important to be realistic about the job model and the kind of person for whom you are looking.

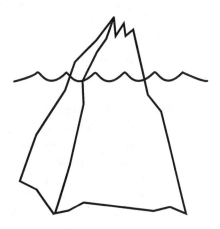

When building your practice team, take into account the value of the individual to the practice goals and client service. When a staff member is hired, keep the interview notes (with strengths highlighted). When that paraprofessional or professional departs the practice, stop and evaluate the reason in light of the strengths that were recorded at hiring. If you changed the role that the person was to fill, then look into a mirror for the real cause of the high staff turnover. I hope you can change your management behavior for the sake of the remaining team members.

Developing a Successful Staff

Five Steps to Developing a Successful Staff

Five steps to staff success—another sure-fire management system that will work for everyone, right? Wrong! There are a few premises that must be shared to have the seven steps work for you. First, you must believe the team can outperform the individual, yourself included. Next, you need to accept that the most significant variable in the practice is your staff, since they are about the only controllable variable that exists. Third, it must be safe to delegate and hold others responsible, while understanding that at first mistakes not only will occur but are also signs of progress, of moving to new, unknown horizons. Lastly, you must be willing to pay for personal success, in accolades, feedback, and payroll. If these "limitations" are not a problem for your comfort zone of management, read on.

Play to Strengths
You hire a person because he or she has traits, skills, or experience that you feel will help the practice. Use people for their strengths; let them worry about their weaknesses. By "use," I don't mean manipulate. We often underutilize our staff or assign a new staff member to menial tasks that provide no esteem or personal gratification.

If the new employee has expectations that are not met on the job, disharmony occurs. We set up those expectations in job descriptions, interviews, and peer performance yet do not realize the disservice that occurs when we underutilize the person after the 90-day orientation. Challenge employees quarterly to reach beyond their comfort zones to develop a stronger team. Regardless, hold them accountable for results, not processes.

Train—Train—Train
In 1890, completion of the eighth grade represented an adequate education. To be really educated in 1930 took a high school diploma; in the 1950s, any college degree; and in the 1970s, a master's degree. The simple fact is education is continuous. You must create an atmosphere that encourages continuing education and a system that supports it on a regular basis. Do not let continuing education become a voluntary program. Demand it; fund it; then share the excitement it creates.

Give Feedback

Whether it be good news or bad, feedback that is immediate is a valuable tool; if it's delayed, it detracts.

Performance appraisals should never hold a surprise concerning the past. If they do, the manager failed to give regular and timely feedback.

In my experience, a performance self-appraisal program will benefit 80 to 90 percent of the staff and will make the process rewarding instead of painful. If your existing program pleases that many, don't change. If not, consider this alternative: quarterly goal setting (management by objective), planning, and joint review of how expectations are met. The good news is that 90 percent of the staff will rate themselves at the same level or lower than their supervisor would. This allows the supervisor to be a hero and to stroke their egos by raising their ratings on specific issues.

Deal with Comfort Issues

Handle personal problems as they arise. Or, at a minimum, facilitate resolution with an outside agency. I don't know who started the rumor that personal problems were not a concern of management, but they could not have had any real life experience with veterinary practices. As a team, we must care for each other and understand that some form of unhappiness will enter every person's life. How flexible is your practice in assisting staff members to work out their problems?

The new buzzword is employee assistance programs (EAP); these include a full scope of services, such as income tax assistance, professional counseling, alcohol rehab, substance abuse counseling, day care centers, health club membership, pretax healthcare accounts, and benefits administration. The range of options is almost limitless.

Employees don't forget organizations that stand by them, just as clients don't forget practices that help with grief counseling at times of pet loss. Programs encouraging employee loyalty started in the United States, went to Japan at the height of unionization, and have now begun to return to the United States. It is interesting to note that the organizations that are the most supportive have the best return on investments. They save money because of lower costs, fewer claims, reduced turnover, and team efforts.

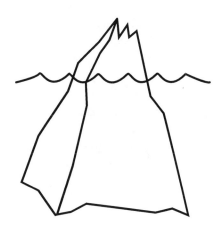

Define Consequences Clearly

The fifth and final step to developing a successful staff is to evaluate the behavioral consequences in your practice. The truism that drives this concept is "Behavior that is reinforced, rewarded, and recognized is likely to be repeated; that which is not is likely to end or diminish gradually."

Given this premise, most practices inappropriately reward. When sick and absent, you get paid. When you injure yourself, you get paid. When you hurt a client or patient, the insurance pays for your mistake. If you retire, the government pays. It is interesting to note that we have developed systems that reward the behaviors that don't help the organization.

We need to acknowledge wellness, attendance, and positive participation. Some practices have replaced sick days with wellness days, with unused balances going to year-end bonuses. I have helped some practices group vacation days, sick days, and continuing education (CE) days into a single category of "paid personal days," to be used at the employee's discretion.

Do you have standards for performance that are as clearly defined as those for nonperformance? I assisted one practice to establish a form of way-to-go certificates for perfect time cards in a pay period as well as for other good behavior. A specific number of the certificates could then be redeemed for a U.S. Savings Bond (double the face value for purchase price). What about quarterly award banquets or hero-of-the-month recognition for that employee who best saved the day during the month? Review your recognition systems for results, not for how much you pay out.

Remember there can be no tolerance of mediocrity. The minimum level of performance in any practice must be competency. I see only these levels of veterinary care performance: needs training, competent, able to train others. Any other terminology avoids the consequences. People are not stupid, and they will meet expectations if clearly stated or will seek other employment.

If we use staff for their strengths, train them to remain current, provide meaningful feedback, confront issues head-on, and have established procedures to reward good behavior as well as correct shortfalls, we can then look for successful staff development. We won't prevent all problems, but we will facilitate their resolution.

We must be professional yet friendly, direct but flexible, understanding but with high expectations. Rewards need to outweigh the bad news. If we don't promote professional advocacy, the outcome is guaranteed—practice mismanagement.

Perspective Management

In the quest for greater productivity, we often mistake assumptions for fact, then wonder why our systems do not work. One of these assumptions is that our perspectives of problems and issues are accurate. This is not necessarily so.

Each staff member has a view on where the practice is going and how it should get there. If this perspective does not match the boss's or if the boss's perception of the staff is off-target, then it will be difficult for the practice to succeed. Hospital directors need to keep a few key principles in mind:

1. Never step into the trap of playing the role of parent, priest, pal, or psychiatrist. These roles belong to others. The hospital director's responsibility is to be the leader in a staff member's professional life—nothing more.

2. Many hospital directors don't have time left for managing after they have finished the list of extraneous tasks they assign to themselves. No hospital director should assume the responsibility of operating a human relations agency. A director cannot provide a comprehensive social work program that will make everyone feel loved, protected, and adored.

3. Responsibility for staff members' success or failure lies with them, not with the practice. A hospital director must learn this lesson: "You cannot be responsible *for* people. However, by necessity, you must be responsible *to* people."

4. When hospital directors become responsible for people, they overstep managerial and leadership boundaries and adopt those individuals. A good rule to follow is *"Build on the strengths, let the weaknesses be a personal quest of the individual."* The perspective of building on the positive will keep the practice on track.

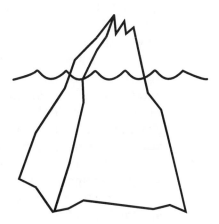

5. The perspective that everyone knows his or her job is false. Knowledge about veterinary medicine doubles

every 18 to 24 months. Training is a must in today's competitive world, and the practice leader who pursues continuing education opportunities for every staff member on a recurring basis will have the strategic edge.

The training a practice provides influences the staff's perspectives. For example, in clinical program training, the "first client" who must believe in the program is the staff member who must talk to the clients. The rest of the staff must support the program with equal vigor, but the real client must *hear* the belief in the voice of that first client.

Marketing and the Staff: Internal Promotions

In this time of increased competition, the natural urge of a practice is to increase its marketing effort. The problem is most bonded clients will not respond to external marketing, but the poor clients will. Clients who respond to coupon and discount offers will not be loyal to any practice. Coupon clients will follow the bargain of the moment. However, there is a form of marketing that a veterinary practice can and should be doing. It is called *internal promotion*.

Rhetoric

The term "marketing" carries a lot of negative baggage in the veterinary profession. We have clients, not customers! We have a social contract based on the trust clients feel when they walk through the front door. Coupon practices often live on new clients and talk of gross rather than net. Most quality practices live on return clients. These practices spend five to six times less money on return clients than they do attracting new clients. Veterinary healthcare cannot be a buyer beware relationship. In fact, the only thing a veterinary practice should ever *sell* is peace of mind. The client is then *allowed to buy* all else.

To make the client aware of what is being offered, the terminology must be clear. A healthcare provider should only speak in terms of need and not use confusing phrases that include "recommend," "should," or "it would be best that." For effective internal promotions (marketing), a client should be given two yes options, such as "We can do this dental today or make Fluffy an appointment for a week or two. Which would you prefer?" In fact, when a healthcare provider states a need, the room should become silent until the client speaks. If the silence must be broken after a "need" statement, the only phrase that should be used is "Is this the level of care you want for Fluffy?"

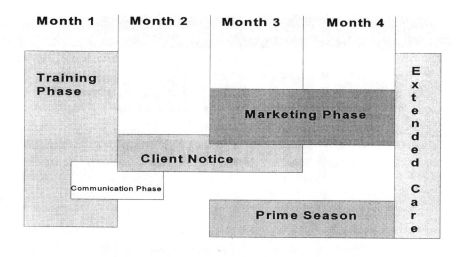

Fig. 2.1. Promotional plan flow chart.

Training

Figure 2.1, which is from Vol. 2 of *Building the Successful Veterinary Practice,* reflects the phases of an effective internal promotion (marketing) program. It starts with *training.* It always starts with training. Not only must the doctors train the staff, the technicians must train receptionists, and receptionists must train technicians. Narratives, values, expectations, and standards of excellence must be shared within the practice team. Every practice team member must be persuaded that the program can, and should, be done. As staff try it (practical application), they need to be coached, and the appropriate behavior needs to be reinforced. Once they have been trained, persuaded, and coached, then, and only then, should the program be delegated to them.

As the training phase ends, the communication phase starts: How can we share the value of this program with clients? The initial client test phases and client reactions must be discussed at a team meeting and the narratives modified and rehearsed again; then another test must be done. As the initial client communication phase is initiated, expect that adjustments will be needed. This will ensure that the practice staff admit prob-

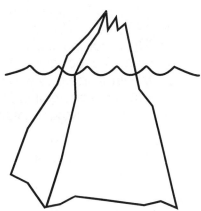

lems and offer feedback. Celebrate the feedback and adjustments. Reward innovation and improvements.

The marketing phase occurs in the prime season. For instance, when the January and February slowdown occurs in companion animal practices, tag on to the dental month and promote an alternative to the holiday bad breath complaints. In the spring and fall, look to teeth floating to get the horse winterized or summerized. The canine geriatric programs don't work well, but a fall arthritis program gets good results if we tell clients to watch for slower movement in their pets (the natural effect of the cooling fall weather).

The extended care is for preferred clients. Your practice can define preferred clients any way you want, but the usual definition is clients who keep their animals protected according to the veterinarian's wellness recommendations. Preferred clients are allowed access to all special programs for an additional 30 days to ensure they get the total benefit of being practice patrons.

Figure 2.1 illustrates a four-month practice plan, but programs will operate concurrently. For example, training for the March-April heartworm and parasite prevention program starts during the January-February dental marketing promotions. The internal promotion system for the entire year must be aligned with community needs, practice philosophy, and standards of care embraced by the practice team. Team members should know what the training plan will be in April so they can drop hints to clients during the practice encounters earlier in the year (e.g., house training and canine behavior management to support the schedule for May-June puppy classes). Planning for success is not as easy as celebrating success, but planning must come first, so just do it and then celebrate!

The Small Practice

Many small practices get through their early years with buddy-buddy nonmanagement, and it works well. When the practice grows and new staff come onto the team, the perspectives are unclear, and the managerial direction cannot be found. Everyone tells the new arrival what to do in the buddy-buddy small practice. If the veterinarian finally sits in the driver's seat out of necessity, some staff rebel because they feel demoted.

Too many small veterinary practices try to function as a family rather than a business. While this is very effective for the buddy-buddy nonmanagement needs of staff made up of family members or family-plus-one, the effectiveness starts to deteriorate when more nonfamily member staff are added because the practice lacks the foundation for organized expansion. The training program must become formalized and planned, or confusion will become the standard. In confused practices, a series of painful and costly adjustments of perspectives have to be endured by all, from the staff on the front line to the bankers with the capital.

Hard Decisions

No one ever said effective management was easy, and leadership is more difficult than management. If leadership were easy, then anyone could be a leader, and new theories wouldn't be formulated every few years, consultants wouldn't be needed, and management would earn the same wages as the paid staff. But leadership in management is painful, especially when developing the mental toughness and single standard required to keep everything in perspective, for self and others.

Leadership in management requires not only tough decisions regarding the staff but also tougher decisions that affect personal discipline and sometimes family or friends. In the life of every hospital director there comes a day when he or she cannot play the buddy. Perspectives must be addressed, training and retraining may be required, and perceptions must be managed to meet the goals and objectives of the practice. Success is just that close, or that far away, depending on your perspective.

Promote Your Practice by Promoting Your Staff

How you treat your staff members is how they will treat your clients.

—*Dr. T. E. Cat*

In most cases, a multiveterinarian practice is only as good as the staff who support it. Most practice owners fail to expend enough time and energy to develop their healthcare delivery team. The staff have the majority of the client contact time, and their belief in the practice and in the services is what impacts the perceptions of the pet owner. Good assistants are an investment. By nurturing them, practice efficiency can be improved, staff turnover can be decreased, and client return rates can be increased. The investment starts with decent pay, benefits, and a work en-

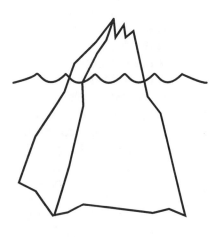

vironment that promotes pride in self and the practice, but there are other alternatives that could economically promote morale and motivation.

Primary Motivators

One of the simplest motivators (the most important in Europe, according to recent research presented at the American College of Healthcare Executives) is a sense of belonging. The concept of belonging to the veterinary healthcare delivery team starts with a feeling of trust. It is enhanced with the practice logo and name on a hat or shirt. Some practices even buy windbreakers with the practice name and staff member's first name embroidered on the jacket. Does the practice celebrate birthdays? When I practiced in Rheinpfalz, Germany, everyone got a birthday letter and a day off with pay (I tried to make it the one next to the closest weekend so the staff member had an extended weekend holiday break). Is there a changeable letter staff board in the reception area with everybody's name and title proudly displayed? Do tenured staff members get business cards with their names and titles printed on them? These are a few ideas for promoting a sense of belonging.

Another important motivator, yet often overlooked by veterinarians, is recognition. This is the primary motivator of American healthcare workers and is number two on the European list. Recognition must be timely and specific. "You did great today" does not convey real recognition, while "I liked the way you handled Mr. Rossi" is very specific and will likely cause the behavior to be repeated. The more recognition given to staff members, the more those achievements will recur. Conveying job satisfaction is often as simple as the veterinarian patting a team member on the back and saying thanks. Recognition does not require an expensive program, but it can make staff veterinarians stretch their own comfort zones when looking for those small successes.

A third motivator in both the United States and Europe is responsibility. When a doctor says, "I trust you to do this task," it is a form of recognition. When the veterinarian does the work technicians were trained to do, it has a negative impact. The staff do not feel trusted to do what they are willing and able to do. In the more progressive leadership situations, responsibility involves making specific staff members accountable for specific outcomes. *Accountability* means continuous improvement is expected, and *outcome* refers to the final result, not the procedure. Most practices see accountability for specific outcomes as

$$\text{input} \longrightarrow \text{process} \longrightarrow \text{output}$$
$$\textit{sick animal} \quad \textit{healthcare/cure} \quad \textit{well patient}$$

This simple model does not promote accountability since the process must be totally directed or controlled by the veterinarian. In the true health-care model, the delivery system is

input ——→ process ——→ output ——→ outcome
*sick animal   healthcare/cured   well patient   happy client
                                                           happy staff
                                                           net profit*

With this new perspective, the staff has many areas of responsibility or accountability when it comes to ensuring client satisfaction. The only thing we really sell is peace of mind. The client is allowed to buy from the list of alternatives offered to meet the patient's or provider's needs. Pride in performance comes from exceeding the expectations of the doctor or the client, as well as from helping the patient. This pride in performance and service promotes greater practice efficiency, more client-centered efforts, and a happier team environment.

The independence associated with the charge to become accountable for the outcome rather than just perform step-by-step processes allows fresh approaches to be brought into the practice. In fact, who knows more about reception needs than the receptionist? Yet in America, where appointments are the rule, most practices do not allow the reception staff to even design an appointment log to meet practice needs. The doctor just buys a standard book and makes the staff write in the margins. Responsibility also means staff members can grow to the point where they work outside the supervision and knowledge of the practice owner. At this point, the practice generally begins to grow faster.

Other Motivators

Training is always a form of recognition, but whether it be negative or positive is the choice of the trainer. No two veterinary practices are alike. You will seldom find a new staff member who understands all the habits of the practice and doctor, so there are a few steps to follow:

1. Determine the specific practice needs, set the performance standards, and ensure each staff member understands the same set of expectations.

2. Careful, patient training in the precise details required by the practice owner and veterinarians will yield far

better results and greater profits than just expecting staff to learn on the job.

3. Don't skimp on time. The orientation to the practice (observing one day in each operational area plus one day with each doctor) should occur before training. Some practices have a 90-day probationary period to allow all training to occur before the hiring decision is finalized.

4. Initial introduction to duties should be done verbally, followed by written job descriptions, protocols, and procedures to reinforce the explanation. This veterinary practice introduction must include an awareness of the overlap and interdependence between the various staff members and doctors on the healthcare delivery team.

5. In busy practices, be willing to pay overtime to the trainer and/or new staff member to get the training done right the first time.

6. Most importantly, after the training is complete and once it is made very clear what a staff member is to do, let him or her do it without interference. Interference stifles initiative and creativity. It is very damaging to a new staff member's morale.

The most successful motivators appear to be associated with training and education—promoting personal growth in knowledge and skills. There are alternatives within this area:

1. Underwrite educational expenses, including seminars, meetings, journal subscriptions, and other profession-specific activities. By reimbursing part of the enrollment expenses and then offering a significant reimbursement of the balance upon successful completion, attendance and participation is promoted. Never be satisfied with an existing knowledge level. The field of knowledge in the veterinary profession is doubling every seven years (you will be 50 percent out-of-date in seven years).

2. Encourage membership in professional organizations, veterinary-based as well as groups like the Delta Society (an international group dedicated to the study of the human-animal bond within the environment) and other animal-related professional organizations.

3. Give a staff member "the rest of the day off with pay" as a thank-you for past performance. This easy motivator is often overlooked. You could even eliminate sick days and roll all existing paid days off into "personal days." This rewards the healthy staff member, not the sick one.

4. Monetary recognition makes an impact, but consider how it is given. If there is a need for extra cash at home, attach a large denomination bill to a letter that specifically thanks the person for his or her effort (the practice assumes the tax liability). If there isn't a dire cash need, gift certificates at a special store allow a shopping spree that offers a dual reward when given as "Take the rest of the day off with pay and go shopping on me!" Giving an end-of-year bonus before Christmas, no matter how small, is always a welcomed surprise.

Each staff member on the team supports the professional, or veterinarian. In most other healthcare fields, this person has the title paraprofessional. It should be the same in veterinary medicine. After some of the above concepts have been accepted as practice philosophy, share the practice's pride in the staff members who accept their new roles by promoting their expertise and dedication to the clients and to colleagues. There is nothing wrong with introducing a staff member who specializes in nutritional counseling, dental hygiene, or behavior management as a paraprofessional.

Regardless of what you do, there are many ways to improve staff morale and motivation. It is equally easy to let things slide and take your assistants for granted. Yet with a little thought and a few actions—by sincerely attempting to understand the characteristics and needs of each person on the team and by recognizing each person's strengths and utilizing them as resources within the practice—every practice can improve. The side effects of prolonged tenure, increased pride, and daily enjoyment of the practice will be the value-added benefit of promoting the veterinary healthcare team. The team's pride will promote the practice because, in very simple terms, "When pride is the input, quality is the outcome because clients perceive pride as quality."

Stimulating Productivity

Productivity is the only effective answer to
recessions and inflation.
—Dr. T. E. Cat

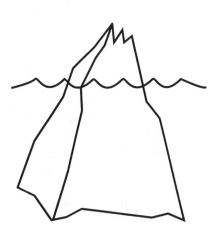

In the past, increasing practice liquidity meant cutting costs. Last decade, most veterinary practices got their costs under control. Most all healthy veterinary practices now keep their monthly operational expenses to below 50 percent of the monthly revenues (less the major variables of DVM monies, rent, and ROI). The better managed, mature practices keep the operational expenses hovering around the 40 percent of revenues mark (less the DVM monies, rent, and ROI).

The Carrot or the Stick?

Stimulating productivity is different than behavior management. We have all heard of the carrot-or-stick approach to horse training or the two-by-four approach of getting a mule's attention before training. While these ideas are entrenched in our heritage, they are not generally used. Rather, alternatives are sought that will serve the same purpose. When trying to increase productivity, you need to look at alternatives to the traditional reward and punishment programs of your practice. Look again at the behavior principle

Behavior that is reinforced, rewarded, or recognized
is likely to be repeated.

or the inverse,

Behavior that is not reinforced, rewarded, or recognized
is likely to end or diminish gradually.

To better understand what is meant by the traditional reward and punishment factors, look at what most employers have rewarded in the past:

✓If you are sick and stay home from work, you get paid.
✓If you have an accident and injure yourself, you get paid.
✓If you damage property, someone else will pay for it.
✓If you don't support the team, the boss will talk to you about compromises.

Vacation pay, sick pay, insurance support, and a lot of other traditional benefits are not bad. They should be in place, but we should be innovative in their delivery. What happens to people who have never gotten sick or to those who always support the team or to those who offer more good suggestions than anyone else? These types are seldom recognized. We take many hours of our precious time to address the problem employee, but the solid performer is taken for granted. We sure send some funny signals to our staff if our performance appraisal system is based on the past without any form of mutual goals or objectives in place. The single most frequent comment that employees write on attitude surveys is this: "The only time you hear anything from management is when you do something wrong."

The Wishing Method

We often wish our practice staff were more efficient, our protocols more streamlined, and our documentation requirements reduced. We wish for these things but do not take the time to train staff. We only want to delegate the tasks! As healthcare professionals, we tend to focus on equipment and technologies and miss the major opportunity.

Productive work environments call for unleashing the natural pride (and thus motivation) of our paraprofessional teams. Motivation is usually diminished because staff members do not feel valued, respected, or supported. The multiple standards embraced by the veterinarians cause staff members to do their jobs without regard to the practice's needs. Staff find it difficult to work to their full potential since no one seems to care or recognize their efforts. They wish for better days but do not want to take the chance of asking for them.

Healthcare research indicates that 60 percent of the paraprofessionals believe they are significantly underutilized. Those hundreds of ideas on how to improve the practice never get passed up because no one listens. If managers do listen, most often the idea is defined out of existence. The reception staff know what clients are saying, but the technician staff know what the patients need. To make a decision, veterinarians feel they must choose a side. Most veterinarians wish the arguments would go away. However, if a veterinarian did not take a side, but rather caused interaction to occur, and reacted positively and proactively to the team compromise, the challenges would go away. Don't you wish it was this easy?

Making It Happen

A productive work environment is created by instituting a process to surface staff concerns and to deal with the issues that are on people's minds. This process takes time and perseverance. However, this is the shortest route to increasing productivity. For practices that equate productivity with increased gross, there are only three ways to increase the gross income: (1) get more clients, (2) charge more for the existing services, or (3) get the client to return more often each year. Each of these three meth-

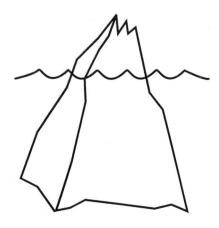

ods will cause geometric growth of a practice, but concurrently using two or more causes exponential growth. Regardless of which of the three income growth ideas is selected, the operational secret for success in a veterinary practice is working through the people on the staff. A seven-step model has been used successfully in other healthcare settings:

Step 1. Commitment

The example set by the leadership is critical; then you need to ignite the effort with someone who will launch the process and make it happen. The champion of the process must be a team member who has successfully recommended a change, has been appropriately recognized, and has been encouraged to try something else. All of these "has" factors are based on the assumption that the leadership will grab every opportunity to reinforce the new attitude by recognizing and rewarding innovation.

Step 2. Assessment

Once you select a productivity initiative, learn the real issues from the staff. Ask them directly for alternatives. Try some early questions, like "What is it like for you to work here?" or "What does it take to make you feel you have succeeded?" or "What is going well?" followed by "What are your concerns?" or "What could help you do your job better?" As the issues emerge, listen, take notes, and wear your rhino skin. Defensive replies or justifications will kill the process.

Step 3. Vision

Staff members usually know what is wrong with the practice, and they talk endlessly among themselves about it. Listening to complaints does not produce the same results as listening to alternatives. The initial effort to change should include building a vision statement with the staff. They need to understand and support where the effort is going. A vision is not a new set of numbers, a new graph, or even new job descriptions. A vision relates to pride and motivation, to a belief in contribution and belonging, to a feeling of being valued. Envisioning the workplace of tomorrow can have a profound impact on the team, especially if that vision is shared and agreed upon. When all the horses pull toward the same target on the horizon, the power is something to behold.

Step 4. Informational data

Traditional barriers must be recognized, and these are frequently based on computer data. However, dialogue with staff has to be based on people's feelings, not on electronically manipulated figures. An understanding must be shared and the concerns of the staff must be heard and prioritized, even if the feelings have been under the table for years. If the emperor is not wearing clothes, someone must make it an issue. There is no such thing as a dead issue if it still elicits staff concern. Using staff ideas as informational data is a good way to acknowledge that the dead issues still exist and have merit.

Step 5. Recommendations

Once the most critical issues have been elevated to the top of the list, alternatives and options must be sought. The two key questions that seem safe are "What are some of the small actions that will actually help our system work better?" and "Can we change or improve the system in some way that is ongoing rather than come up with one-time-only ideas?" It is important that the alternatives are a series of small, incremental steps that can be accomplished in days or just a few weeks. A comprehensive overhaul will seldom get off the ground in a veterinary practice. There is never enough time to stop and do a total rework or install a new system.

Step 6. Change

The ability to launch a change with enthusiasm is far easier than keeping the new process going with a positive attitude. The inevitable resistance to change derails even the best plans unless there is someone who will keep putting the engine back on track. In the average veterinary practice, once a change has been implemented, priorities shift, and no one seems to care that the new initiatives have been forgotten. Every time the leadership puts the innovation system back on track, the vision will become that much clearer for the staff.

Step 7. Recognition

When firing up the innovation engine, not only are the idea people important to recognize, but the doers are too. Every great idea requires others in the practice to support it, to nurture the new process, and to refine it until the desired outcome is achieved. Immediate recognition is critical to fuel an innovation engine. A comment, a staff meeting mention, a quiet gift of a movie gift certificate, or similar actions are very effective. People are eager to do their jobs well, but they don't want just a productivity program. They want to be valued and appreciated.

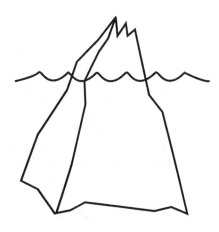

Pressure to work harder and faster is not recognition. Giving them credit for the new outcomes will be.

The Never-Ending Story

The dog dragon of storybook fame comes alive to children who believe in it. (I found a very similar dog dragon painted on the bedroom ceiling of Mad King Ludwig's castle in Bavaria—so who was being innovative?) The vision of the practice can have the same life, one of fairy-tale proportions. Visions can grow but should not be seen as impossible to meet. Staff efforts should not become never-ending pursuits of an undefined dream. The measurement of success must be established at the start so completion will be clearly recognized. This way, shortfalls are still successes since they at least moved the practice away from the inertia of the status quo. There are no magic wands in this kingdom, only leaders with a vision that can be shared. The results are dazzling to those who have come to believe that it is impossible to change the system, but they are not magic.

Whether they admit it or not, veterinary practices hire people to solve problems. Those who are hired to do jobs are never great successes. The job description is the minimum standard of performance. Staff members must search for the maximum levels based on their strengths and attitudes. Performance plans have replaced performance appraisals. A veterinary practice that has all "10" employees is a practice without a vision, without anywhere else to grow. This satisfaction with the status quo also defines a practice that is going to die soon. Stasis is death, in medicine as well as practice management.

The paradigm shift is to work smarter, not harder. The work week is less than 40 hours, not more than 60. The goal of the client-centered model is to have satisfied clients coming back more often. This is smarter. The goal of the discount practice is to steal more clients more often, creating volume, so the practice works harder. This a short-term income producer but seldom a career satisfier. The Band-Aid approach to productivity is over. It is time to make the commitment to the practice team for change as it sees it.

Recognizing Productivity

In some practices where I have consulted, there have been some unique payments, recognitions, or rewards established. In most all practices, good words from the veterinarian are underutilized. There is a practice in Delaware that provides an award certificate for error-free work (such as a month without a time card error) or for significant practice contributions. When a specific number of certificates are amassed, they can be redeemed for a U.S. Savings Bond. There is a practice in Tampa that has grouped vacation days, sick days, and CE days into a single category of paid time off called "personal days." The number of total days varies with ownership, tenure, and position. A Michigan practice provides contests almost monthly to allow staff members a rewardable way to help the practice grow.

The inverse of these rewards is negative reinforcement, when the manager uses most all available energy to fight fires, beat staff into submission, and threaten their employment status. Sounds dumb, doesn't it? Negative reinforcement happens in very subtle ways in some practices. Look at the interactions that currently occur in your practice. Are they guarded? Are things the way they always have been because that's the way you've wanted it? These are indications that negative reinforcement has occurred in the past and no one wants to face the dragon again. There are alternatives.

Veterinary Extenders

Veterinarians produce the gross; the staff produce the net!
—Dr. T. E. Cat

A veterinary extender allows the primary provider (the veterinarian) a greater amount of time to see patients and talk to clients. The veterinary extender may be a person or a thing. Sometimes veterinary extenders provide ancillary services such as nutritional or behavior counseling. At other times they relieve the veterinarian of business work, like inventory control or supervision of the animal caretaker team. The veterinary extender may be a well-designed form, a very friendly computer program, or, sometimes, a volunteer.

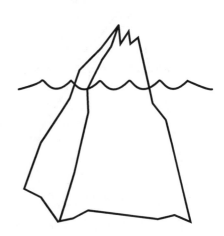

For contemporary veterinary technicians, animal caretakers, and receptionists, this veterinary extender caregiver model is offered as the essence of shared practice success. The focus of this system of caregiving is simply skilled veterinary healthcare professionals working in the best interest of the patient. For example, technicians once checked the patient into the facility, performed the bathing, and then discharged the patient to a pleased client.

Now the practice receptionist admits and discharges while the kennel person (animal caretaker) gives the bath. The modern technician has assumed the supplemental role (veterinary extender) in health screening (physical examination) of the patient at admission and client education during the healthcare program.

An analogy of this veterinary extender caregiver model is based on the sandbox theory. Typically, children play alone in their sandboxes. In this model, however, all the kids in the neighborhood come to play in one giant sandbox, and together they create a unique and special sand castle. If someone tries to knock the sand castle over or if it starts to rain, the kids in the sandbox rally to shore it up and make it even stronger. This is the secret to an effective practice team of veterinary healthcare professionals. Each person assumes he or she can make a difference in the quality care of the patient, client, and community.

The Veterinary Extender Caregiver Model

The veterinary extender caregiver model brings together professionals and paraprofessionals with diverse skills, talents, and abilities. Together they address issues at the very essence of veterinary medical practice: "How can we do more for the community we serve? How can we share and exchange our talents, knowledge, and skills to help our patients, to support the veterinarian(s), but, most importantly, to assist our clients in their stewardship of our patients?" Look at Figure 2.2 for the interrelationships that need to be understood.

Many practice owners fail to understand that the central issue for their staff is often not compensation and benefits but, rather, concern about clients, patient care, and their environment. Practice staff are justifiably angry because many veterinarians prevent them from practicing the professions for which they were educated and trained. Practice owners must realize that in this way their staff are no different from other professionals. If their needs go unmet, they will regress. Stymied in their search for self-actualization, they will look for self-esteem. If self-esteem is elusive, they will seek autonomy. With no autonomy, they will meet social needs through negative communications with coworkers. And if the social structure breaks down, they will pursue the basics of living: wages, salary, and benefits. In the process they may get what they want, but they will lose sight of why they initially entered veterinary healthcare: to care for the patients and support the clients. This is often the cause for burnout.

Although every veterinary practice may not be willing to create the equivalent of a full veterinary extender caregiver model, each could benefit from increased participation of staff members. In facilitating any innovation, keep in mind the following factors:

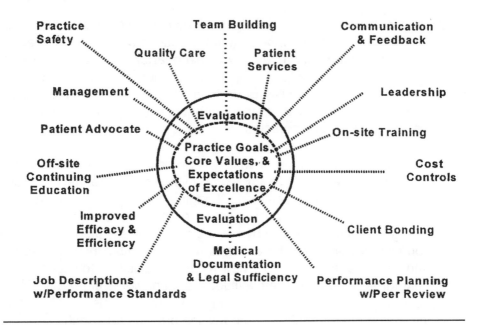

Fig. 2.2. Veterinary extender caregiver model.

1. Prepare for a mixed reaction. Some staff members may not enjoy an expanded role with its increased accountability and responsibility. Change is not comfortable; in fact, change requires discomfort, not with the practice but with specific habits that no longer benefit the practice. Although some staff members are dynamos, others may just want to work eight hours and go home. Change requires too much effort for the latter group. Realize that, although some staff may want to stay with your practice forever, others will invariably leave.

2. Work on your own attitude and the example you set in daily activities. Banish negative stereotypes. All too often supervisors or veterinarians make comments like "What do they know? They're only receptionists" or "Technicians just want to be junior veterinarians." What most all staff members really want is to be all they can be within the practice. Many veterinary practices have yet to create an environment where that can happen, but your practice could be among the first.

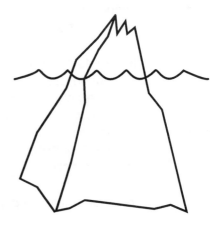

3. Practice owners must be willing to spend time with the staff and other veterinarians. At least once a month, practice owners should attend a community veterinary meeting. At least quarterly, the lead technician and receptionist should participate in an appropriate CE experience outside the practice facility. Equally as often, supervisors and leaders should talk to each staff member about his or her concerns—professional, practice, and personal.

4. Be willing to invest time in what will probably become a three-year process. Remember that traditional systems of veterinary practice have been around for decades. Changing habits is a slow, incremental process where a specific policy or procedure is identified for change. It is first defrosted by making people dissatisfied with the action or outcome, then the action is remolded into a new procedure, and then it is refrozen into a new habit by repetition. To expect a 24-hour turnaround in policies, attitudes, or behavior is unrealistic. Have patience and be prepared for delays, postponements, and backsliding during the maturation of the revised practice approach.

5. Encourage a positive attitude toward failure. Help staff understand that if a program or effort fails to meet expectations they have still gained by the learning process. They can never be expected to stumble unless they try to move forward. They can still revitalize the practice by building on current strengths and positive attitudes. Allow people to verbalize their concerns in a nonthreatening atmosphere.

6. Get employed veterinarians to buy into the program. Talk to the veterinarians in terms of patient welfare, client bonding, and returns to the practice. Help them understand that a good veterinary extender allows them to have more patient hands-on time and, thus, greater productivity. The benefits of increased productivity will make them commit to the program.

7. Share information routinely—including key financial reports. Shared information does not need to be the bottom line of a financial report, but rather, it needs to be related to what each person could affect in daily operations. If the staff feel important and involved, they will look for ways to improve the systems they can affect. Good leaders look for these opportunities to share accountability. Decreased costs and increased services will enhance the practice's fiscal position.

8. Focus on quality of care. The client is more than a customer, and the

pet is more than just a patient. Quality care centers on client needs, patient wellness, and perceptions of satisfaction. Continuous quality improvement (CQI) is based on encouraging each staff member's pride in his or her level of contribution as well as promoting the client's perception of quality care. You don't need to educate most staff members about quality patient care—just give them an environment where they can practice patient advocacy and concerned client communications. The veterinary extender must be allowed to make changes within established guidelines for the benefit of the practice without having to ask permission. The top quality healthcare practice will attract and retain clients looking for top quality veterinary services for their pets.

Application of the Veterinary Extender Caregiver Model

The first step in the application of the veterinary extender caregiver model (Fig. 2.2) is to administer the charge-out test (Fig. 2.3). This is as much a calibration of the leadership as it is of the staff members, so give it to every staff member during your next staff meeting (veterinarians must participate). It is to be completed independently within five minutes using the routine resources available in the practice.

Once everyone does the exercise, discuss it in a staff meeting. If the staff aren't able to agree on a figure, this supports the need for a better veterinary extender caregiver program in the practice. Lost income can be recaptured. Ask for the rationale of the charges, pro or con; then ask what the best level of care should be at your practice. Do not be surprised if the range of charge-out test results among the staff is over $200.

Pride and Quality and Veterinary Extenders

Another important application principle of the veterinary extender caregiver model that cannot be forgotten is that when pride goes into healthcare delivery then quality is what comes out. Quality is based on the perceptions of the client; it is not a simple input into the process of healthcare delivery. Continuous quality improvement occurs when the practice leadership releases control of the process and sets clear ex-

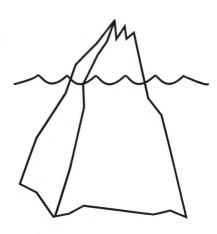

PLEASE CHARGE OUT THIS CASE IMMEDIATELY:

No doctor is in the hospital and you MUST give an estimate to this person. Her one-year-old, 25-pound beagle mix was hit by a car six days ago. Everything is now okay, except that the pet needs to have a major organ removed (right kidney) to lead a normal life. The vaccinations are current, and the fecal was negative. The pet is on year-round heartworm preventative and the Difil test was negative. The surgery will take about one hour, and the dog can be discharged 48 hours after the surgery. Because we are using isoflurane gas anesthesia, there is only a very slight anesthetic risk. The client is settling the previous account right now, so how much do you expect the total surgical care bill to be at discharge?

$ _____

Fig. 2.3. Charge-out test.

pectations of outcomes. It is when the practice leadership assigns accountability rather than tasks. It occurs when leaders encourage change for the betterment of the practice, by every staff member, without telling staff members, "We don't do it that way."

Some practices have adopted core values instead of job descriptions, such as PRIDE or I CARE, which represent:

P—patience	I—the important person in the formula
R—respect	C—the client comes first
I—innovation	A—action is what the client wants
D—dedication	R—respect for self and others
E—excellence	E—excellence is competency

There are many variations to the use of veterinary extenders. Some practices require three staff per on-duty veterinarian while other practices have one staff member for two veterinarians. The latter case never allows the development of a veterinary extender approach to healthcare delivery. The bottom line for veterinary extenders in the 1990s is simply: "If it is to be, it is up to me."

Leading Your Team

The objective of leadership is to accomplish the mission in the minimum
time and with the maximum balance of individual needs.
—Dr. T. E. Cat

Profit-based performance standards require effective leadership to make them work as positive motivators. The ultimate objective of leadership in any organization is always the successful accomplishment of the goals and objectives of that organization. Catanzaro & Associates has defined the ultimate veterinary hospital management objective as follows:

To ensure quality healthcare delivery for every patient presented, with an acceptable rate of fiscal value return, and adequate quality of life for the practice and its staff, while establishing a clearly defined and client-perceived veterinary services market niche in the community.

But we would prefer to say it as follows (it's easier for others to remember): A leader's hospital management objective is to foster

- Delivery of quality healthcare
- Proper remuneration of provider and facility
- A clear community market niche
- Staff member pride and quality of life

In striving to achieve this goal, the leader must accept full personal responsibility for all of his or her decisions and must continually assess the practice environment. Continuous quality improvement (CQI) requires that every member of the staff is accountable for the daily activities and takes pride in the tasks performed; the client perceives the outcome of staff efforts as quality care. Using profit-based performance standards is one method for recognizing the staff's contribution to the hospital's CQI program.

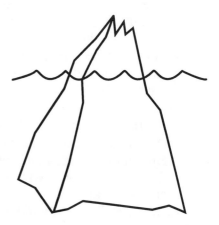

Styles of Leadership

Too often leaders focus their efforts on short-range goals at the unnecessary expense of their subordinates (the team is subordinate to the leader but does not need to be made to feel that way). In the long run this can be detrimental to both the staff and the practice. Effective leadership is accomplishing the mission with a minimum expenditure of personal time and effort and an appropriate balance between practice, staff, and individual needs and goals.

Leadership ability becomes increasingly important as the practice team expands. When the practice becomes a multipractitioner healthcare delivery system, leadership becomes a prerequisite for team building and success. While there are many styles of leadership—shades of grey in the spectrum of good approaches that must vary with the situation—most all can be classed as either directive or nondirective leadership methods. The directive leader tells the staff exactly what to do and lets them know who is the boss. Group members have the secure feeling of knowing exactly what is expected of them. Nondirective leaders seek the opinions of team members, consult with them in planning and decision making, and sometimes, on nonhealthcare issues, even put ideas to a democratic vote.

Match Leadership Styles to the Context

Neither approach is appropriate at all times. In general, directive styles will be more appropriate in lifesaving situations and with beginner-level employees, and a more participative style will be better for practice management situations and with professional and paraprofessional associates.

Summarizing research, models, and theories developed by a variety of social scientists, Dr. Chemers, of Claremont McKenna College, gives this advice: "If your subordinates do not have the knowledge necessary to perform the task, or if their attitude is such that they lack commitment to the goal at hand, a directive approach is warranted." The most common example of this situation is the chemotherapeutic regimen for a patient, where the drug, dose, and duration and administration are dictated by the veterinarian.

Of course, even the best veterinarian doesn't always have a clear picture of what the most desirable course of treatment should be. You may need a colleague's perspective or the staff's ability to provide subjective information on the case or client; here, participation is called for. When a veterinarian is nondirective, it is more likely that the team members' intellectual abilities, years of practical experience, or technical capabilities will contribute to a task. This is especially true for challenges in practice management that deal with client bonding or improving productivity.

The participative style has some important bonuses. It makes team members feel autonomous—a proven motivator for many personality types—and it gives them the opportunity to develop their skills. In deciding between the two schools of leadership, also consider the bottom line—can subordinates be expected to energetically implement a management decision if they didn't participate in making it?

A Compatible Fit

If one style or the other feels uncomfortable to you, don't be surprised. Many theories assume that any person can be equally adept at any behavior; this just isn't the way it is. A considerable body of research shows that leaders have personal styles that they are more comfortable with and that they habitually use.

If you are the type who is very concerned about relationships, harmony, and acceptance by the staff, you will lean toward the participative style. It places greater emphasis on morale. If it is important that people like you, you will have difficulty with the directive style of leadership. On the other hand, if you need order and have a strong desire to accomplish a task as efficiently as possible, you will most likely favor the directive approach.

Knowing which end of the spectrum is preferred by your colleagues can help you work with them more successfully. If you are the associate and the practice owner is highly directive, you can depersonalize and defuse most situations instead of taking her personality as a personal affront. More importantly, if two veterinarians are both directive in style, there will be conflict about whose directions are best. Both want an orderly practice environment—but based on their own order. If both veterinarians are participative in nature, they may want to avoid conflict so much that they don't control problems and, therefore, waste a lot of time.

If staff recognize their own inclinations and the leadership style of the boss, problems can be identified before they reach an impasse. But regardless of style, the secret of good leadership is to communicate effectively. This means that information is given *and* received in each exchange.

The Filters

Information is processed at various levels of understanding based on the mind-set of the listener. Every person has these filters. Some of the more common used by practice leaders include

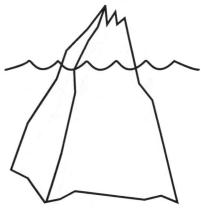

■ What the leader believes he or she "heard," either verbally or in writing. Clarification is seldom discussed.

■ What the leader believes the staff should know for their own good or to protect the practice.

■ What the leader believes the staff want to hear, regardless of the practice needs or environmental situation.

■ What the leader thinks should be toned down or built up for the benefit of the receiver. Facts are mediated.

■ What the leader's values and attitudes do to the information—the bias of prejudice and personal ethics.

■ What stress the leader is operating under, at home or in the practice.

■ What importance the leader attaches to the information and the leader's perception of the validity of perceptions other than his or her own.

■ What the leader feels at the moment that the information is being received or when passing the information to others.

When we consider the filters that information must pass through at each level, it is clear why there is distortion, dilution, or total lack of communication. Do not misunderstand: it is the leader's job to overtly filter messages in order to clarify them and indicate their importance. The leader, however, should not allow personal feelings and stresses to filter communications inappropriately or covertly.

The downward flow of information has the practices' seal of approval behind it. On the other hand, feedback is critical to ensure communication has occurred; remember, both the giving and getting of information is essential for effective team communications. The average veterinary healthcare delivery team has filters that often interfere with meaningful feedback. Some common filters that staff members apply to upward communications are

■ The notion that any opinion in opposition to the boss's idea is negative thinking and therefore bad.

■ The notion that practice teams always gripe, and you should only worry when they don't.

■ The belief that the information is unimportant and that the originator does not have the big picture in mind.

■ The belief that the veterinarian is not interested in the paraprofessional perception.

■ The belief that you will get into trouble for passing along this type of observation or information.

■ The belief that the information will reflect adversely on you, your ability, or the staff effort.

■ The belief that the practice manager/ownership only wants to be told the good things and not the bad.

Please do not think that all filters are bad. Some filters serve a useful purpose. You should try to solve problems, or when addressing a problem, offer at least two alternative solutions. You need to take the appropriate action, try the best alternatives, and pass on the significant information. Whining is not constructive communication. The acid test for staff is to ask whether or not they would need or like to have the information if they were in the leadership position.

The Bridge

Some guidelines for communicating more effectively with either style of leadership are

- Keep it short, simple, and direct.
- Word your questions so that they will elicit a yes response; your position is then associated with the positive.
- Suit your message to the audience.
- Use words like "let's" to automatically associate yourself with the team.
- Use a story or anecdote as a window. Construct a vivid scenario of "what if" or "when" to make the team imagine the events already occurring.
- Use words like "right" or "truth" to put your position on the positive side of a debate.
- Know when not to speak. A dramatic pause after a particularly important point will stress your sincerity. It also allows you to evaluate the reception. If negotiating, present your case then leave in silence.

Improving your own communication skills so that you can practice varying leadership styles is only smart business. Select those problems you can improve and do your best. Do not spend great amounts of time fretting over things you cannot influence; it makes for a far better practice environment.

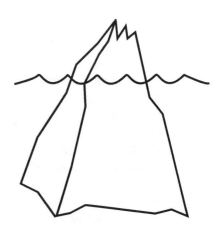

Through an awareness of the filters and barriers in the practice communication systems, a leader can decide which communication system can be used, how to reduce the effects of the filters, and where to look should breakdowns occur. Good communication does not just happen—it must be developed and maintained by the team leader.

An important facet of any leader's responsibility for developing and maintaining effective communications is that of daily coaching and counseling. The veterinary healthcare team wants to be better; it wants to give the best to the clients and patients. Communication is the most significant means of influencing team members' behavior, their self-worth, and their participation in the practice's goals and objectives.

What Is a Hospital Administrator?

As the only Board-certified veterinarian in the American College of Healthcare Executives, my perspective may be slanted. I believe there is a difference between being a hospital, practice, or business manager and being a healthcare administrator (see *Veterinary Forum,* February 1995, p. 63). Managers deal with programs and process; administrators deal with outcomes, getting things done through other people, and the use of leadership skills.

Ten Areas of Concern for Hospital Administrators

As a consultant, and as a healthcare administrator, I've found that the old school of veterinary practitioners demands a job description. I consider a *job description* simply as the minimum standards of training required during the introductory period of employment. I prefer *job standards,* which are the outcome expectations of those who hire a person. Because practices have different expectations, job standards for a specific position are not always going to be the same, but the areas of interest are. For example, I see 11 major areas of professional development required for any veterinary hospital administrator:

Organization
Governance
Organization arrangements
Bioethics and practice values
Planning
Marketing
Human resources
Financial assessment
Facility planning
Professional education
Quality improvement

The reference text *The Well-Managed Community Hospital,* by John Griffith, provides a complete integrated overview of the environment and activities of a well-managed facility. There is not a similar comprehensive reference in veterinary medicine, although there are many references (and quick-fix gimmicks) that are a mile wide and an inch deep. For the purposes of any veterinary medical practice, completing the practice-specific points that follow should provide the job description/job standards required for effective middle management leadership and facility operations.

Organization

Interpret the practice's role with respect to health service values.

Define the organization's mission and practice philosophy.

Ensure effective admission and disposition of patients and their stewards.

Develop the criteria for evaluation of management efforts.

Evaluate the internal policies and procedures relative to the practice goals and objectives.

Report organizational performance to the owners.

Develop criteria to evaluate owner performance toward practice and staff.

Assess the impact of change on the motivation of the work groups in the practice.

Set standards of action required to achieve goals.

Governance

Be able to explain in detail the difference between policy and implementation and accept that the role of the board or ownership is to set the standards.

Explain the implementation requirements for the practice's annual budget and long-term (three- to five-year) plan.

Develop an organizational structure, delineating accountabilities and authority, which meets the practice's mission.

Formulate and promulgate policies and procedures that concern professional responsibilities of the practice.

Assist to define and establish a set of core values that translate practice theory into action at the staff operational level.

Provide orientation and direction for professional members of staff.

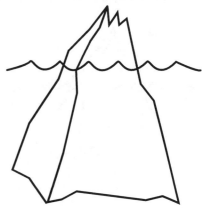

Organization arrangements

Identify presence and function of other veterinary providers in area.

Develop informal cooperative relationships with other veterinary providers, agencies, and specialists.

Negotiate formal affiliations (contracts).

Ensure a continuity of care and establish and maintain a medical record accountability system.

Develop informal linkages with educational institutions.

Establish appropriate linkages with various advocacy groups.

Assess the technology impact and potentials for the practice.

Ensure organizational arrangements for legal counsel.

Ensure organizational arrangements for internal control audits.

Identify and evaluate state-of-the-art computer technology.

Establish information system (computer) support program.

Ensure integrated systems and data gathering occur within the practice.

Bioethics and practice values

Assess current demographic impact of community on practice.

Review clinical ethical issues and initiate appropriate action.

Establish and ensure a routine peer review of veterinary healthcare delivery is conducted and documented, in the practice and by medical records audit.

Identify and respond to conflict of interest situations.

Keep informed of criteria and standards of veterinary healthcare delivery.

Review business ethical issues and initiate appropriate action.

Understand and implement grief and stress counseling for clients and staff.

Develop and promote policies, procedures, and practices that balance the needs of management, providers, clients, and patients.

Interpret medical/professional staff conduct on behalf of the practice.

Planning

Implement the organization's mission statement.

Establish an internal and external communications plan.

Plan for timely client access, effective examination room utilization, efficient surgical suite obligation, and staff-doctor-client-patient interactions.

Analyze community needs and demands for veterinary services.

Ensure a supply and replacement program is developed with multiple vendors to maintain an appropriate cost of goods sold.

Assess the needs and initiate the training programs required to enhance the capabilities of the staff and practice.

Ensure consistency between long-range and short-range goals.

Assess the economic resources available for daily operations.

Eliminate or modify the unproductive programs based on sociological, economical, and political considerations.

Involve all team members in planning to achieve goals and objectives.

Evaluate how eliminating a program would impact the practice's continued success and survival.

Identify measures by which practice performance can be quantified.

Assess human resource strengths and availabilities for the practice.

Marketing

Assess use of public relations, marketing, and advertising to meet practice goals and objectives.

Differentiate between internal promotions and external marketing.

Establish the appropriate internal and external promotion plans to meet the wants and needs of the practice, providers, and clients.

Assess the cost benefit of specific programs compared with client benefit and staff benefit assessment methodologies.

Select multiple methods to measure client satisfaction with the practice.

Identify and initiate target-marketing efforts and promotions to established and/or potential clients.

Determine methods to increase client and patient return rates and to track successful implementation.

Human resources

Establish a human resource philosophy to motivate team members.

Promote human resource philosophy through practice structure and policies.

Evaluate alternative compensation and benefit programs.

Develop criteria for effective staff benefits and for a responsibilities manual.

Identify and assign outcome areas of accountability, ensuring authority and responsibility are delegated to achieve success.

Evaluate performance and productivity at all levels.

Assess manpower needs, including skills assessment and shift demands.

Ensure consistency between practice policies and existing laws.

Plan for effective practice scheduling of staff members.

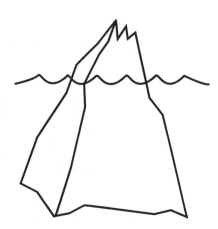

Promote teamwork and motivation within the staff members.

Arbitrate matters of dispute between staff members to achieve proper operational effectiveness.

Develop an outplacement program for terminated staff members.

Financial assessment

Establish a capital equipment demand list and provide it to ownership.

Implement an industry-based Chart of Accounts and financial accounting system (see Vol. 2, *Building the Successful Veterinary Practice: Programs and Procedures,* Appendix F).

Plan program-based budgets to reflect income-to-expense balance required for quality patient care, liquidity, and client bonding.

Develop workload forecasts, cash flow projections, and program-based needs for practice success in sequential periods of operation.

Respond to external forces that diminish the practice's assets.

Develop a system to ensure confidentiality of business records is maintained.

Utilize trend analysis and fiscal factors to assess profitability of programs, people, and the practice.

Develop business plans to enhance new program planning and implementation.

Evaluate the operating budget relative to practice goals and actuals.

Initiate variance analysis as needed to ensure negative trends can be addressed and reversed in a timely manner.

Develop an integrated system to control accounts receivable.

Utilize cost-finding methods to assist in decision making.

Recommend rate structures and fee schedules that marry the philosophy of ownership with the wants and needs of clients and staff.

Facility planning

Develop a master site plan based on long-range practice goals.

Plan for proper maintenance of the physical facility and equipment.

Determine alternative flow patterns that enhance productivity, performance, and client friendliness.

Develop the program to purchase capital expense and facility improvements required to increase effectiveness.

Ensure proper procedures for storage and movement of drugs, supplies, and equipment.

Implement the required procedures and policies for making minor alterations and improvements.

Professional education

Establish an appropriate, monthly, in-service continuing education program for staff and providers.

Review the professional trends and schedule program-enhancing experiences outside the facility.

Ensure appropriate literature is available and reviewed in a timely manner.

Assess the impact of technology on existing programs and policies; ensure changes are initiated to provide liability protection and enhanced care.

Encourage staff to participate in continuing education and promote literature review discussions to evaluate comprehension and implementation.

Motivate professionals and paraprofessionals by appealing to their sense of pride and professionalism.

Quality assessment/improvement

Review quality assessment methodologies and develop a team methodology to initiate improvements.

Implement, evaluate, and monitor the risk management program (OSHA, safety, radiation protection, zoonotic disease, etc.).

Ensure each client's and each staff member's dignity and safety.

Analyze various reports relating to quality improvement to ensure desired outcomes are being achieved/pursued.

Ensure adequacy, confidentiality, and availability of all patient/client care documentation.

Select methods to measure the quality of services being provided.

Be aware of all regulatory requirements (DEA, FDA, EPA, OSHA, etc.) and ensure appropriate programs are established to protect staff and practice.

Develop a program for managers and providers to independently improve the quality of services and care being offered and delivered.

Establish an ongoing patient advocacy and client relations feedback program.

Discuss identified problems in quality standards, such as in patient care or facility safety, with medical/professional staff and reach commitments for outcome changes.

Implement a quality improvement process within the practice.

Be prepared to participate with respective staff members in taking corrective actions required for quality improvements.

Provide reports to the governing body on results of quality improvements.

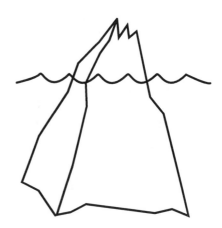

The Rest of the Story

In all of the above rhetoric, a quality administrator is still not defined. We can use all the phrases made famous by consultants:

No one on the staff will care how much the administrator knows
until they know how much the administrator cares.

Managers will take credit and give blame
while leaders give credit and take the blame.

The respect required to be effective is born in caring.

The L in quality stands for leadership.

Leaders can only establish the environment for motivation; the good team
members find the key within themselves.

They all say the same thing but in different ways: leadership is the common key to veterinary healthcare administration. Innovation and creativity are most often stifled by managers and enhanced by leaders. So the final elements of any job description/job standard needs to end with two clauses:

Meet the challenge—solve the problem!

Challenge the system—make the improvement!

Application Exercise

As stated in the Introduction, mind mapping is an excellent technique not only for generating ideas but also for developing intuitive capabilities. Use the iceberg ideas you have added on the odd-numbered pages and the concepts you have drawn from this chapter to expand the following mind map.

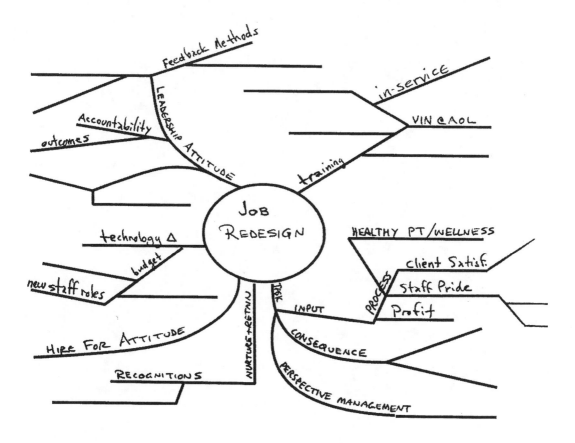

CHAPTER THREE

Creative Client Power-Up

Treat the customer as an appreciating asset.
—Tom Peters

Innovation and creativity in client service are far more than sending a coupon or offering a discount. In fact, at the current profit level of most practices, for every 5 percent discount provided a client, an additional 20 percent of business must be acquired by the veterinary practice. Practices must see the world through the eyes and feelings of the client, must be client centered while becoming better patient advocates, and, most importantly, must be so consistent that everyone in the practices will be in harmony with the quality and continuity of care discussed in Volume 2 of *Building the Successful Veterinary Practice*.

Most every veterinary practice worries about internal controls accounting for receipts, drugs, and tangible property, as well as cash controls accounting for the pennies a day it may lose. But most clients are worth thousands of dollars, and practices ignore their protection. For a client, the process of selecting a veterinary practice may take a matter of minutes or it may take many months, but the practice bond can be broken in seconds. In Appendix F, the medical record assessment forms utilized during my on-site practice consultations have been included for practice self-evaluation. Granted, any form of peer review of medical records is generally painful, but if used as a commitment to improve the continuity and quality of care, the hurt becomes profitable, improving attitudes as well as net income.

Creating the Client Bond

The First Step—Awareness

Obviously, before a consumer can become a client, he or she must be aware of the facility's existence and of the need to seek services. It is often assumed that this step can be accomplished by a Yellow Pages ad and an outdoor sign, yet many pet-owning households in the catchment area may be unaware of all the practices within a 15-minute drive of their home. Once they find a practice, a tour of the facility is seldom offered, so they are unaware of the high-tech, personalized philosophy of the practice. What is your practice's new client:practice tour ratio? Have you placed behind-the-scenes scrapbooks in each examination room to allow clients to have a picture tour (pictures of people helping animals, not just equipment waiting to be used) while they are waiting? Are pictures labeled, identifying the patient, the procedure being conducted, and the staff member's name, then updated regularly to show new practice programs in action?

Image—Beginning of the Bond

The client acquires knowledge about a veterinary practice in a variety of ways, the most common being through nonverbal awareness (smells, sounds, visual cues, etc.) of the environment, followed by the examination room communications. What sets your practice apart from the other practices in the community? What is special? What is different? If the answers are a crowded reception area, lack of parking, repeatedly being put on hold, or other negative factors, your image needs immediate attention. One way a practice can improve its public image is through active community leadership; worthy causes are the sweetest and most cost-effective since media coverage of a socially conscious practice is usually free.

The consumer has a set of values fostered by television, magazines, books, and other media sources, and these values drive the consumer's image of your practice, either positive or negative. Word of mouth impacts this image, as will the practice environment, so a practice must be concerned about the perception of quality in all its activities. Step back and look at your practice and the word-of-mouth programs. For example, how are referrals handled? Is appropriate client behavior being rewarded (e.g., outreach thank you programs)?

Knowledge Is Key

Typically, clients begin patronizing a clinic in increments. The first step for most clients is preventive or emergency care, then, later, health maintenance care. As clients form a practice loyalty, the practice finds it easier to market the full scope of services needed by each pet, horse, or production animal owned. Once a preference is formed, the client will act upon it when the need arises. The veterinary practice will share knowledge in many ways, from tailored handouts for the community (a practice directory with contact points for animal control, animal services available, poison control, etc.) to glossy vendor promotions to audio-visual systems designed to increase community awareness of the scope of services available.

Have you looked at those brochures in your mailbox? Those from organizations trying to get money for their charities? They hook the audience, not through rules and policy, but by evoking the readers' emotions and listing reasons to subscribe. Quality is the most important facet of a practice's image. In one-on-one sessions, staff members' pride is what influences clients' perception of quality, but there are many other parameters, and their significance varies by region or community.

Research by a human healthcare national research firm in 131 major cities of the United States showed a high variability within six basic factors affecting quality perceptions. Six of those cities are shown in Table 3.1. It is interesting that care was seldom a significant factor unless an exclusively female population was surveyed, and for this group, in many localities, equipment was less important and care was the primary concern.

Advocation—Becoming a Believer

If the practice experience meets or exceeds expectations, consumers typically become advocates. They will be regular users of facility services, will make over-the-counter purchases, and will simply make word-of-mouth recommendations to potential clients. However, if the experience is negative because of delays, unfriendly staff, an unexpected triple-digit bill, a rushed veterinarian, or a host of other variables, the client will change preferences and a patient (or patients) will be lost. Consider forming a Council of Clients, a dozen clients and their significant others who come to a dessert meeting once a quarter and provide insight on needed services, perceptions of quality or care, and changes needed to increase their utilization of the practice's services (more on this later in the chapter).

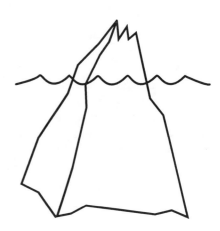

How we approach a community or prac-

Table 3.1. Consumer perception of quality factors

City	DVM	Staff	Care	Service	Equipment	Image
Chicago				X	X	X
Akron		X		X	X	
Cincinnati	X					X
Pittsburgh	X				X	X
Indianapolis				X	X	
Denver		X	X			

tice population is dependent on practice philosophy, professional interrelationships, and the target population (elderly, multiple-cat households, owners of geriatric dogs, etc.). Regardless of which targeting strategies are used or which target population is in the primary catchment area (location is always critical), the promotional messages must be carefully developed, and the whole team must be involved in this process. A smart practice will strive for multiple client visits per year, spreading out the costs but increasing the total access to practice services.

Segregation of Function

One of the most critical elements of any internal quality control program is the *segregation of function.* This simply means one person does not have total control of an asset (e.g., the person counting the money at the end of the day is not the one who closes out the computer record; the two people then compare the two totals).

SEGREGATION OF FUNCTION — INTERNAL CONTROLS

**The same parameter applies to the client as an asset;
no one person must control that asset.**

The client must encounter a team of caring providers, from the receptionist to the outpatient nurse (technician) to the veterinarian who recommends an *internal referral* to the other practice doctor for collaboration on more involved cases. Even the use of external specialists indicates a team approach; it symbolizes the practice's desire to deliver the best care possible. Regardless of the Monday morning syndrome, in most every veterinary practice the phone is an underutilized tool for client communication (for getting *and* giving information).

When a client misses an appointment, who should call him or her and how soon? The message can be simple, such as "The doctor and I missed you *and Fluffy* today (yesterday, this week, this month, etc.). Is everything okay at your house?" With vaccination reminders (which should first be sent at the eleventh month and, instead of listing specific vaccination codes, should state the client actions needed), if a practice really cared, a client's nonresponse would prompt a receptionist's call within 72 hours of the expiration of protection.

The nursing staff (some people call them "technicians," but clients better understand the term "nurse") have an important role also. In the case of a postsurgery, the nurse anesthetist (technician) should call the client when the animal recovers from anesthesia to ensure the client understands the discharge planning coordination; this should be followed three to four days later by another call from the same surgical nurse (technician), "We know you *and Fluffy* will be in next week for the suture removal, but the doctor and I just wanted to reassure you that if any of your family members had any questions about *Fluffy's* procedure or recovery process we are here for you."

The outpatient nurse should call clients two weeks after a flea control program is initiated because that is the next time a treatment cycle is indicated, a nutritional counselor should call a client after 20 cans of a case are utilized to offer to order another case of prescription diet before it runs out, the dental hygiene nurse should call three weeks after a dental care "deferral" to check on gum condition ("red equals pain, so we must get the tooth out"), and an outpatient technician should call 10 days into a 21-day cystitis treatment with a caring message, such as "We know *Fluffy* is only half way through the treatment program we prescribed, and that you and *Fluffy* will be in next week for the recheck, but the doctor and I just wanted to reassure you that if any of your family members had any questions about *Fluffy's* treatment or recovery process, we are here for you." If some of these narratives sound familiar, it is simply because caring is a consistent message we want to convey and we know it requires from 6 to 16 contacts (this varies based on client awareness, beliefs, and knowledge) to make clients respond to a new healthcare need.

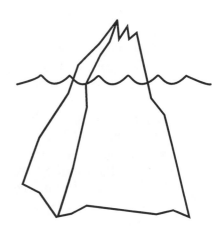

The doctor will retain 20 to 30 percent of

the primary callbacks, due to specialized information or client-promised diagnostic feedback requirements. However, the team approach will help diversify the handling of incoming client calls, since clients will become used to the team approach in healthcare monitoring and the telephone follow-ups. Any practice with more than two doctors on duty should consider the use of a telephone receptionist to increase the routing of incoming calls to the appropriate person, to increase the responsiveness to clients making appointments and the calling of clients who missed appointments, and to decrease the disruptions for the front desk team, who should be receiving clients with a helpful smile.

Veterinary practice clients are an appreciating asset, so you must appreciate them, and let them know how much! American clients hate to be sold anything, but they usually enjoy the opportunity to buy. A caring veterinary practice team *only* sells peace of mind—everything else the client is allowed to buy. Clients are stewards of living creatures and deserve a caring and knowledgeable veterinary healthcare team to help them in this commitment. Clients will become better assets as they are nurtured by the team, and better clients are seen more often. Clients who are seen multiple times per year will seldom follow the newspaper ad or go to a discount clinic, unless the practice bond is broken by an uncaring team. This is how an appreciating asset is developed. Try it—your team will like it and so will your clients.

Customer versus Client

The magic formula that successful businesses have discovered
is to treat customers like guests and employees like people.
—Tom Peters

Many new, hungry, uninformed veterinarians start their practice careers by competing in price, rather than differentiating their practices by meeting unmet community needs. But to survive, veterinarians must center on the challenge of the marketplace and the perceptions of their clients.

- When the client enters the front door of a veterinary practice, it is the beginning of a social contract.
- The client is expecting the practice healthcare team to meet his or her expectations and to provide the appropriate care needed by the pet.
- The practice team expects the client to give an accurate history, to care for the pet in a humane manner, and to compensate the practice for the services delivered.

■ Better practices always try to exceed the client's expectations, since this determines the client's perception of the quality of a practice.

The Business Approach

Traditionally in business, customers have alternatives based on elasticity of demand. This elasticity is based mostly on price. If the price is too high, customers will shop for a bargain, delay purchase, select a cheaper alternative, or not purchase at all. Customers are assumed to be informed and able to substitute, delay, or go without. However, for a client with an animal suffering from an acute illness, severe pain, or trauma, price may not dominate in the decision process. This client has lost the power to bargain, delay, or go without; the demand is inelastic when it comes to preservation of life or relief from undue suffering. The only thing we sell in veterinary healthcare is peace of mind.

Considering the *peace of mind* charter, there appears to be a paradox when veterinary clients are called our customers. Some practices endorse the customer approach with coupons and bait-and-switch tactics, such as a low-cost surgery offer, which includes vaccinations, anesthesia, parasite testing, dental offerings, and similar services being hard sold to clients when they arrive. At the other end of the scale, some practices do not even participate in phone price quotes; they require a patient examination before determining the anesthetic risk.

Other traditional goals of business have been to maximize profit or market share and, secondarily, to satisfy customer wants. The veterinary hospital has always sought to provide quality care for patients in need. In healthcare, quality comes first, proper compensation to the provider and facility come second, and developing a community market niche is the third business priority. There may be conceptual and factual dangers in trying to provide services dependent upon profit motives rather than delivering the quality care expected based on the veterinarian's oath. Profit follows a quality healthcare delivery episode, but it does not follow when the client perceives he or she was "sold" something that wasn't really needed! In the latter case, the client often decides to go elsewhere the next time. Remember the first rule, *the front door must swing* before any money can be made.

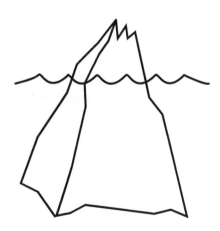

Marketing, creativity, public relations, innovation, point of purchase displays, patient needs versus consumer wants, and merchandising are ubiquitous terms and phrases in veterinary healthcare literature. Topics like patient advocacy, peer review, and quality assurance appear infrequently in our literature, yet they remain the ethical foundations of veterinary practice management programs. There is an unwritten social contract between society (or the community) and the veterinary medical establishment to minister to individual and herd health needs. In return for the benefits we provide, society accords the veterinary health professionals substantial independence, prestige, and monetary rewards, although these monies seem to be harder to find lately. This social contract is unique to healthcare, but it is in jeopardy in today's competitive market. We must recognize this trend and develop mechanisms to preserve the covenant and social purpose of veterinary medicine.

No client can be worse than no client.

In veterinary medicine, the term "client" may be becoming overshadowed by "customer" or "consumer," at least in our recent marketing-focused literature. The difference between a veterinary client and a customer is that the social and moral responsibility to a client should be sacrosanct. This is the belief that caused most of us to enter veterinary medicine.

A customer is defined by the ability to bargain for commodities. A business exists to provide commodities and is successful if it remains competitive in a dynamic free enterprise system.

A veterinary practice exists to provide services to meet the social contract between society and the healthcare system, which is based on caring, treating, curing, preventing pain, and saving animal life.

Following are the differences between customers and veterinary clients:

In business	In healthcare
The customer can say no and go elsewhere for a quote.	The client feels at the mercy of the healthcare provider.
Most people are there voluntarily.	Wellness concerns force access by the client.

Most people are in a good mood.	Most clients are anxious and scared or feel exposed.
Many people feel they can bargain for a deal.	Most people are panicked about the required costs.
Customers expect to be pampered and served, often by staff members who are inexperienced but try to please.	Clients are often confused by high technology but expect know-how and compassion from the professionals.
Employees must try to be courteous and responsive to the customers' desires, regardless of the demand.	The client must be responsive to the professional's case assessment, while the staff must be safe, accurate, kind, skilled, alert, and much more.

In light of the veterinarian's oath and these concepts about clients, it would appear to be unethical to consider animal owners with pets in pain as customers. Veterinary patients have needs, not wants, so the owners have needs, not wants. Some practices unilaterally determine hospitalization needs and scope of professional services, many times failing to offer needed care for economic reasons. They advise their clients about the minimally adequate healthcare requirements for their pets, then turn around and scheme to market services to them as customers. This seems less than professional to me.

We need to change the exam room approach of veterinarians; they need to become communicators as well as healers. This means we need to change those universities that are turning out unskilled communicators. We may not be able to do this, but we can be accountable for what happens within our sphere of influence. We can improve communication skills within our practices, and sometimes this can be done at the local veterinary medical association level and, for some, at the state or national association level. So look in the mirror—and at the tone set by your practice philosophy:

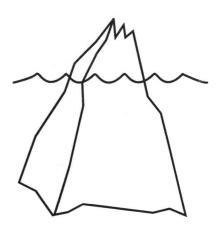

First, accept the responsibility to change your practice style.

Second, start using the word "need" when discussing healthcare, as in "Fluffy needs to be X-rayed for ...," or "We need a blood test to ensure ...," or "I need an ECG to determine ..."

Third, wait for the client's response after any "need" statement. The silence will cause a response; be ready with two options to elicit a yes. "Since you can't do it today, would you like to schedule it for later this week or next week?"

Fourth, record any client waivers or deferrals of "needed" in the medical records, validate the client's feelings immediately (remember, we only sell peace of mind in healthcare), and then tell the client when you need the pet back if there is little or no change.

These four steps uphold the professional side of the social contract. We are stating the needs of the animal (patient advocacy), yet we are respecting the rights of the owner to make a decision (client relations). We are also stating the potential dangers in ignoring the care when we state the need to return (professional ethics). These ideas may be the beginning of a new practice philosophy, if they have not already been integrated into the existing practice style.

Profitable Social Contracts

Whenever a contract is initiated, the goal is for both parties to come out feeling they have been winners. Can you remember the last time a neighbor came home with a new car? Remember the words that were used? In the beginning, he said, "Look at the new car I *bought,* isn't it great!" Later, that month when something started to go wrong, he said, "This is sure a lemon they *sold* me!" When buyers feel they have been sold something, a social contract has been violated. And it is people's feelings that motivate them to refer others to a business.

The key is to get every member of the staff to recognize the social contract and to focus on the clients' feelings. The traditional approach of "treat sick animal, cure animal" is no longer adequate to meet the social contract. Effective veterinary healthcare delivery is now "client arrives with animal, animal is cared for by a team, wellness is restored or protected, client's expectations have been met or exceeded, practice has made some net, and the client is satisfied enough to come back *and* to refer a neighbor." The need to fulfill the expectations, the need to have pride in whatever is done for the pet while the animal is in the practice's care, and the need for a feeling of personal contribution to success are critical elements of the healthcare delivery system. The wise veterinarian promotes participation in meeting these needs.

In the 1990s the trend in the so-called veterinary healthcare industry was to market services and merchandise product lines to customers. This is easily verified by reviewing many of the professional journals. The business customer orientation in the veterinary marketplace caused price competition to increase, decreased salaries and quality of life, and stressed practice survival strategies rather than providing community service. "Consumer beware" has been the veterinary healthcare rule in some communities. The reason for the customer approach is that most veterinarians look for the quick fix to competition pressure.

The Practice Edge

It is the responsibility of each and every veterinarian, technician, business manager, and receptionist to put the practice of veterinary medicine back into perspective. Patient welfare and compassion come first. Patient advocacy and continuity of care must be the motivating forces, and "ethical quality care" the watchwords of the future. We cannot let patient care become secondary to our quest for clients. As I've stated repeatedly, caring veterinary healthcare providers only sell peace of mind!

Quality care can and should differentiate a practice from others within the community. Even in the toughest competitive veterinary marketplaces, low-cost vaccination clinics that offer a doctor's consultation (at a premium price) have about 75 percent of their clients accessing the veterinarian. In other communities, 75 percent of the discounted spay coupon clients have declined to waive presurgical laboratory tests (which means they are paying more than the coupon price). Early human-animal bond research (*The Pet Connection,* CENSHARE, University of Minnesota) showed that 75 percent of families studied considered their pets family members (only a third of those pets were given people status, so don't get carried away). When the pet is a member of the family, clients feel it needs a higher level of concerned care.

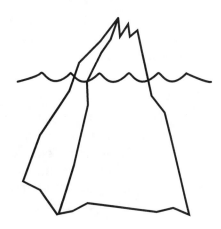

The concept of continuous quality improvement (CQI) gives staff members the latitude to make unilateral changes in their client service, patient care, or personal pride. With CQI, the accountability for better outcomes (client satisfaction and better practice net) is passed down to every staff member. Actualizing this concept does not require a highly skilled practice manager; it requires a caring leader. Are you ready to lead your team into a proactive social contract for success?

A balanced healthcare approach will reinforce our professional position as the guardians of animal health and welfare, and it will ensure the continuity of this healthcare profession. The personal pride and client concern that accompany this approach will provide what we sought when we decided to enter this profession.

The Search for Affordable Value

There are two ways for a fellow to look for adventure; by tearing everything
down or building everything up.
—The Lone Ranger

Veterinary practice is an adventure, and as a consultant, I am always asked to play the role of Tonto. I am there to help, to infuse energy, to offer alternatives for the hospital director to consider (who often feels like the Lone Ranger), but I am not there to lead. I have scouted the canyons of human resource management, followed the peaks and valleys of the cash flow, and faced the temper of the lynch mob (marketing demographics), but all I can do is tell what I've found to the hospital director and hope his or her decision will be to follow my advice.

"There are a million things in this universe you can have,
and there are a million things you can't have. It is no fun
facing that, but that's the way things are," said Captain Kirk.
"Well, then what am I going to do?" asked the ensign.
"Hang on tight ... and survive. Everybody does,"
replied the Captain of the Starship Enterprise.
—Star Trek, "Charlie X"

The veterinary healthcare marketplace is finite. There are limits to the number of pet owners, the number of ranchers, and the animal care dollars available. Tom Peters created the model in Figure 3.1 to illustrate how services must be expanded in a finite market (Fig. 3.1). The center is the core product; the entire model represents the practice's opportunity for innovation and creativity.

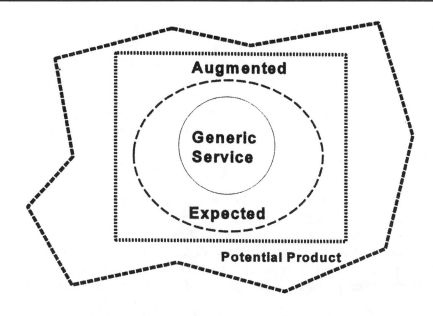

Fig. 3.1. How services are expanded to meet the expectations of the marketplace.

This is not a Star Trek Tribble, soft and chirping. It represents a cold, hard fact of life. The generic services offered in the 1970s gave way to higher expectations and many practices augmenting their services. In mixed and large animal practices, many have stayed within expectations, but care of herd health is often augmented. Over a decade ago, embryo transplant was a potential product, but now it has become an augmenta-

tion. In a specialty service, it is an expectation. Suppliers and vendors responded
to the higher practice expectations by offering value-added products to practices.
Some, like Summit Industries, totally re-
designed their X-ray control panel into the
tabletop to meet the needs of the majority
of the companion animal practitioners.
Companies like Hill's, who used to have a
veterinary-specific allegiance, responded
to the demand from pet food warehouses
and lost some of their augmented market
when they violated the expectations of
some veterinarians. Hill's created a new

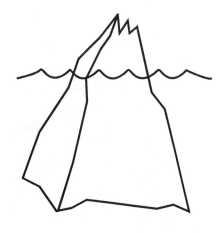

product (HealthBlend) to attempt to give a value-added pet food back to the veterinary practice.

Veterinary practices have responded to increased market expectations in three ways. The first is to "hang on tight ... and survive," in the words of Captain Kirk. These practices try to control expenses and wait out the trend (whatever it is). Some fail as they wait. Practices have closed in numbers not seen before in this profession. For the first time, veterinarians are not recession proof.

A second type of practice has emerged: the couponing competitors. These are the practitioners who target the average client's price sensitivity within the community. It is a shame. Most of them are the lower-end practices, and they are destined to fail. They increase their gross with advertising and couponing but lose their net. Remember, at the average veterinary practice's state of liquidity, a 20 percent discount requires double the access traffic, and a 5 percent discount requires 20 percent more business. Practices cannot survive without liquidity and a significant amount of net.

The third type of practice is the one that has evolved to a higher life form. This type has augmented its expected services, sometimes by bundling potential products and sometimes by unbundling products and allowing the client to ask for the potential product or service. It looks for ways to add value to each encounter, such as spay and neuter credits being amassed with each puppy or kitten vaccination visit. Some practices have started to offer puppy clubs and/or senior clubs to allow animal and human socialization (respectively) at the practice after normal hours. They consider a very inexpensive promotion (value augmentation) when only the salary of one technician is involved.

> *There is only one thing more important than money,*
>
> *and that is getting more money.*
>
> —*Pappy Maverick*

Many practices have fallen into the trap of assessing overhead to every new product or service that comes along. This is called "full absorption" or sometimes "activity-based" cost accounting. Think about the facts. Your practice has an overhead cost, and it is established. It includes virtually everything in the expense column of your profit and loss statement and most of the liabilities on the balance sheet. If you add a new resale product, hang it on the wall and make only a dollar net on each item sold—that is more money than you had before. Sell 100 of those items each month, and your practice has made $100. If the receptionist inventories, orders, and restocks the product on an occasional slack midday period, and the product is kept on top of the cages in the kennel, there has been zero overhead added because of the product line. The $100 is pure net.

The fixed costs are line items such as taxes, rent, insurance, depreciation, legal fees, accounting costs, licensure, dues, maintenance, utilities, telephone, staff salaries, and doctor salaries. Fixed costs often rise in stair-step fashion, with a facility expansion, when a piece of equipment is added, or when staff are added or given a pay raise. On the other hand, drug costs rise as you sell more drugs, so they would be variable costs, as would line items such as supplies, materials, commissions, and freight. As you can see, there are very few true variable costs in a veterinary practice. Fixed and variable costs are compared in Figure 3.2.

There are some who love to allocate floor space as a method of break-even analysis. However, if you did not have the product or service, would the bank reduce the mortgage payment on the floor space? Not likely. Unless you rent out the floor space or equipment to someone else, it is a fixed cost already obligated. It will not be changed by new product lines or services. Once you accept that the overhead of the practice is mostly a fixed cost, then you can proceed to "variable costing," the method to use when changes in costs are dependent upon volume.

"Before I let you go to work, I'd rather see you starve. We'll just have to live on our savings," said Ralph.

To which Alice replied, "That'll carry us through the night, but what will we do in the morning?"
—*The Honeymooners*

Determining what is profit and what is not can be confusing, especially when we start to convert the data to percentages. For instance, profit divided by cost is defined as mark-up percentage, while profit divided by revenue is defined as profit margin percentage. As an illustration, if you buy something for $10 and sell it for $15, there is a $5 profit (variable cost = revenue cost). We all know this, but now the comparison by percentage should be considered:

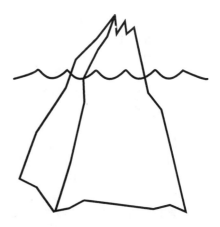

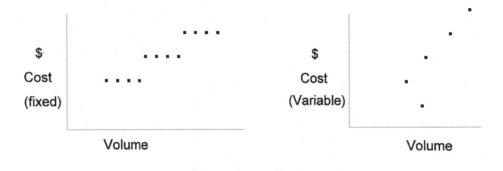

Fig. 3.2. Fixed versus variable costs.

$$\text{Markup} = \frac{\text{Profit}}{\text{Cost}} = 50\% \quad \text{or} \quad \text{Profit margin} = \frac{\text{Profit}}{\text{Revenue}} = 33\%$$

The funny thing is any practice can spend the $5 profit, but very few can spend the 50 percent mark up or the 33 percent margin. The bottom line for most every veterinary practice is to sell services for more than they cost and to sell products for more than they were bought. In this concept, turnover becomes important, but most of the veterinary practices do not pay enough attention to turnover profits. They want drugs in stock when needed, but they have learned not to apply the principle to other practice products (e.g., nutritional items). Inventory turnover is simply the cost of the inventory sold within a period divided by the average inventory in the period. The more turnovers per period, the less money that needs to be invested in the stock on hand. In terms of our previous $5 profit example, whether we sell 5 or 500, the markup or profit margin percentages do not change, but the money in the bank changes from $25 to $2,500. Doesn't this difference make you want to pay attention to turnover? For nutritional products, the distributors usually see 17 to 20 turnovers of their pet food stock per year, and they calculate an active practice has 8 to 12 turnovers per year.

Using national research data received from Hill's, the average revenue from food was 6.7 percent of total hospital revenues, and the average profit as a percentage of total hospital profits was 10.9 percent. In most cases, there were no carrying costs, since the average practice actually sold the products before paying the Hill's bill. For the average practice, what this translated to was an actual $11,408 per year extra revenue from nutritional sales ($661,051 revenues with a saving of $556,769 expenses over the national survey). Yes, inventory management took an average of 3.3 hours per week and about 90 square feet of display and storage space combined, but the work was done in what would otherwise be idle time and the display/storage space had no other income-producing use, so they were both fixed costs. The $11,408 was extra net income in the bank, waiting to be spent.

> *Some men try to climb mountains*
> *others just date them.*
> —*Louie De Palma,* Taxi

How practices address a challenge determines their success or mediocrity. Will the challenge be a motivator, causing the veterinary healthcare team to rise to a new level of understanding about the practice and business of veterinary medicine, or will the staff continue to date around the edges of the challenge, without committing time and effort because they hope the right mountain comes along (or goes away).

The search for an affordable value has become a constant for the client and the practice. The one-stop shopping service is out of financial reach for most practices, especially if they want higher turnover rates. A practice must be able to differentiate itself from others by adding value to each client encounter. Vendors must do the same (watch Hill's for a veterinary-exclusive new product line). Practices are letting clients choose the level of service they desire for their pets (as I originally discussed in 1993 in "Increasing Client Options," *Veterinary Forum*). Other practices offer feline boarding with vertical habitats or playtime for their canine boarders. To be remembered by a first-visit client, practices must do the usual in an unusual manner or deliver the unusual as if it were the usual.

Why a Client Interview?

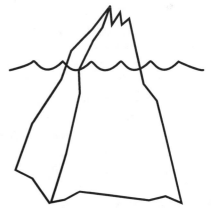

> *Never answer a question, other than an*
> *offer of marriage, by yes or no.*
> —*Susan Chitty*

> *Never ask any question, other than a health*
> *or safety question,*
> *which can be answered by yes or no.*
> —*Dr. T. E. Cat*

Most veterinary practices want clients to come through the front door, have their pets treated, and leave satisfied and ready to return. To encourage them to come back, practices use New Client forms, which include employment information, addresses, phone numbers, and a line where they can sign off that they understand the rules of the practice (see example in Appendix F). This is not friendly, but during the past decade someone convinced veterinary practices that this was professionally appropriate behavior. For the record, I believe in new client information forms. However, I believe the form should be completed through a caring interview by a staff member, rather than just issued to the client on a clipboard.

I prefer the new client interview be done by a technician in the privacy of an examination room. At Westside Animal Clinic, the receptionist team has developed an exceptional client bond by leaving the counter and sitting next to the client in the reception area. Life is a series of perceptions, and the perception of quality is relative to the past perceptions. If we don't understand this, we cannot respond to clients in a manner they perceive as caring, competent, and complete. For instance, four critical bits of information needed from every new client are

1. What has been the client's past experience with veterinarians, if any? (Amount of information the client requested versus that provided, fee sensitivity, inpatient preferences and drop-off needs, time allocated for discussion of concerns, etc.)

2. What is the pet's role in the family? (Is it an assistance animal? Who cares for it? Who is responsible for the healthcare decisions? What type of psychological bond has been formed?)

3. How and why did the new client select this practice? (Why did the client choose us out of the Yellow Pages? Is there someone we can thank for referring the client to us?)

4. Are there any other pets at home (birds, fish, caged mammals, etc.)? Can we put the client on our mailing list when special services or products become available for those species the client has at home?

Answers to these questions are often emotional, and a clipboard will never convey this observation. The follow-up questions, and the clarity provided by a real person, differentiates a practice from others that have an assembly line process. If the pet is their first, clients need a lot of husbandry training from the technician. They also will not intuitively know how skilled the veterinarian is, how complex the diagnostics can be, or how modern veterinary facilities have evolved into wellness healthcare centers.

First-time veterinary clients may also have a severe case of invoice shock unless they become aware of the training, equipment, and services being provided. This information must be shared during the interview process.

The name of the previous practitioner is also important for requesting records, finding out why they left, and letting your colleague know that you have acquired a past client of his or hers. If the client asks, "Why do you want to know?" when asked about a previous veterinarian, tell the client honestly, "We don't want to make the same mistake if at all possible." If the interview reflects an adverse encounter with another practice, share the information with that practice. One dissatisfied client tells about 11 other people, and each of those 11 tell 5 more ... and we only hear from about 10 percent of our dissatisfied clients, so use every encounter to learn as much as possible. You might even learn of a problem in your system and change it before the client can encounter it.

> *There is always an easy solution to every human problem—neat,*
> *plausible and wrong.*
> —*H. L. Mencken*

The above quote is included to remind you *not* to make value judgments about the practice the client left and *not* to tell the client (or others) adverse things about other practices. When you pass on the client's perceptions to his or her former veterinarian, do not try to solve what the client considered a problem because your colleague may not believe it really exists.

> *Every crowd has a silver lining.*
> —*P. T. Barnum*

Most veterinary clients initially select their veterinarian by location. This means in a community without competition you should get about 60 percent of the pet owners when you let them know you have opened a practice. With new veterinarians graduating each year, a community with no competition has become very rare, so we need to look beyond location. In most mature practices in the United States, where we usually average a 20 percent population movement every year, about 10 percent of all transactions each month should be from

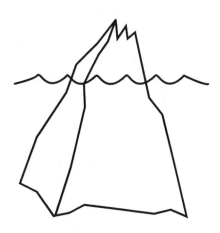

new clients. Less than 10 percent means we are not getting enough of the new trade, and when the new client rate exceeds 15 percent, we are probably not getting the established clients to return often enough. This does not pertain to new practices during their first 6 to 24 months of operation.

One of the most critical bits of information available from a new client is how he or she decided to come to your practice. If no one comes in because of your signage, it probably needs to be upgraded through colors, backlighting, simplification of artwork (or adding some), or the emotional message it conveys. The signage should match the theme of your practice and carry the message. If you want to regularly see dogs, cats, and birds, consider using pictures on the sign to convey this message. If you want fewer cat clients, leave the cat off the logo.

Like Refers Like

In the mature, established practice, we like to see 50 to 60 percent of all new clients coming from word-of-mouth referrals. People tend to refer others who have similar pet values, so finding out who sent the new clients gives you some idea of their expectations. The word-of-mouth practice promotion system can be cultivated or ignored, but as all mothers have learned, "Behavior rewarded is behavior repeated." In most practices, the receptionist team is responsible for initiating a thank you system for those referring new clients, but seldom do the receptionists include another practice brochure or business cards and tell the clients they are for the next neighbor the clients wish to refer. Some practices also add a premium to the thank you note, such as a percentage discount on the next visit, a $10 credit, or, my favorite, tickets to a movie or the zoo. The other nice thing about referred clients is they are generally more forgiving, especially if they catch your practice on a bad day. If their neighbor thinks highly of you, it is worth a second try later.

Some people like to solicit new clients by paying for larger ads in the phone directory. Interestingly, in most communities, less than 10 percent of all new clients are gained through phone listings. Often, people who say they used the Yellow Pages of the phone directory actually were told, "There is a great practice on Main Street," or "Dr. Sato is a great veterinarian," or "Mary said there was a good bird practice in this town." Sometimes the phone listing is used to find the closest veterinarian (if this is so, add a map), the one with emergency hours, or, in today's tightening economy, one who takes charge cards. If any of these become a common reply during new client interviews, capitalize upon the new information next time you place an ad in the Yellow Pages.

IBM always acts as if it were on the verge of losing every client.

—Jacques Maison-Rouge

IBM was an American standard of excellence in the 1980s. The above quote by an IBM executive tells you why. IBM was seldom the most innovative, but it did emphasize service and responsiveness to its clients. This gave it their market edge. By the 1990s it forgot this approach, lost its market niche, and now is having to catch up to the IBM look-alikes. Feeling important is what clients want when they enter a veterinary practice. It is this feeling that makes a new client come back.

> *Four little words sum up what has lifted most successful practices*
> *above the crowd: a little bit more.*
> *They did all that was expected of them and a little bit more.*

Admittedly, the interview process for new clients takes a bit longer than having them fill out new client information forms by themselves, but each client is worth it. The information is invaluable. The bonding that occurs makes a return visit more likely, and every client benefits from the staff's new understanding of client perceptions.

Brochures as a Practice Builder

> *The purpose of a brochure is to make them come through the door!*
> —*Catanzaro & Associates*

The average veterinary practice now has a brochure, usually a piece of trifolded paper that informs the reader about the services available. While this is better than no brochure at all, there is room for improvement. A good brochure builds the practice image while it generates the desired response.

Sell the Image

As discussed in many demographic reports (e.g., *American Demographics* magazine), the client's perception of quality and value in healthcare is based on community, not universal, standards, regardless of what national advertising agencies attempt to sell you. There are many critical factors that may be used to foster an impression of quality care and enhanced services, but most of these will have to be tailored to the veterinary practice's community.

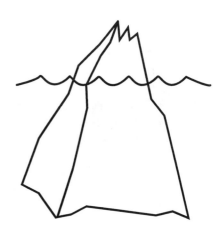

One of the strengths of veterinary practices is the image of caring. The question is how to best differentiate your practice from the growing selection available for clients. Some practices use brochures with cartoons or pictures, some sell the beauty of their ideas, and others combine strong copy with great graphics. Each can create an effective image if the presentation is balanced.

Think of the key phrases that best describe the practice benefits or unique offerings:

- Convenient hours
- Emergencies welcomed
- Feel confident, feel comfortable—join our practice family
- Have a busy schedule? We have evening and weekend hours
- Veterinary-supervised boarding
- Service plus: one stop for all your pet care needs
- Extended evening and weekend hours
- Unaccompanied healthcare for established patients
- Personalized home care
- Comprehensive healthcare for the cat in your life
- Dedicated to alleviating your pet's pain with gentle caring, proven methods, and modern equipment

In some cases, the brochure may offer a value-added reason to use the benefits of the practice:

- Buy one, get one free vaccination program (corona/parvo)
- Quality care doesn't have to be expensive.
- Reduce that breath odor from your pet; visit us for a free predental examination.
- Prevention programs for healthier family pets
- Free introductory pet exams
- Your pet deserves the best without costing the most.
- Bundle services, such as a discounted vaccination series, heartworm/FeLV testing, or health maintenance agreements

Sometimes the reasons appeal to the clients' emotions, as the following examples do:

- Day or night, we are here for your pet.
- Why have our patients been coming back for 20 years?
- Your pet is our family business.
- Not all pets are created equal; neither are veterinarians.
- Friendly staff happy to answer your questions.
- More about the person behind the practice.

- We are problem solvers, especially if your pet is _____ (e.g., hurting, overweight, a problem, etc.).

The lists could continue, but these should provide a few ideas about how a brochure can project the image of quality and caring and differentiate the practice from the competitors.

Common Errors

As a consultant, I've seen many attempts at practice brochures. Most are better than nothing, but many do not reflect the practice's real intent or convey the practice image desired by the ownership. Let's look at a few common errors:

Practice philosophy

A neat subhead, right? Think about when you went to school and how much you liked philosophy classes; your clients are not much different. If you center the subheads on benefits to the pet or owner, then clients will read the paragraph about how your practice philosophy will help them achieve what they want from the practice (e.g., pet wellness).

No differentiation

Since brochures do not do well in bringing new clients through the door, the real question is "Why should a client keep coming to this practice when a new one was built closer to the client's home?" Your written effort should approach this question from many perspectives to ensure clients have many reasons to think your practice offers that something special for their pets and themselves.

No action photos

Photos are excellent to illustrate a point, unless there is no action, no person, or no caring shown; then they are wasted space. Show the caring touch: the technician doing a dental on a cat or the smiling receptionist greeting a client. To have an impact, remember, the person's head in the picture must be at least the size of a dime. Use only "smiling" pets and beware of a background that portrays confusion or disarray. Color photos convey quality. (More on photos later in the chapter.)

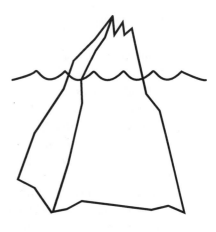

Low-contrast printing

The single-color ink brochures, such as those with blue print and blue photos, are virtually impossible to read. Do not use a soft shade screen for typography, headlines, or photos. Go for the high contrast. Remember, the senior citizen trade increases each day, and this group needs larger (10 point), clearer (no italics, please), modern print styles. A card stock brochure with more than two colors is better than the average brochure used by practices. (More on graphics later in the chapter.)

Pronouns

The term "we" is great in team building, but in client brochures it can be a turnoff. Go for the "you" statements, such as "you'll find ... ," "when you need ... ," "your pet will get ... ," "you can receive ... ," or other statements that include verbs like "discover," "enjoy," "love," "have," "uncover," or other value-related words. This type of approach keeps the interest of the reader, and that is the only reason for a practice brochure.

Professional copy

To the average client, professional text written by the practice staff is usually boring because it is usually too informational. Copy written by many public relations "experts" is no better, since they don't know the clients you want to attract and keep. Such copy is not directed toward a call for action, and it is often dry and unappealing. It is as bad as sending a computerized reminder that "your cat needs FVRCP and FeLV" or "your dog needs DAALPP and Corona." Only veterinary professionals equate this alphabet soup with multivalent vaccines; clients need simple, direct information. Brochures need to have colorful adjectives, action verbs, and vivid word pictures that appeal to the buyer, not the seller.

They Call It Copy—but You Shouldn't

The term "copy" is used to describe the narrative in a brochure, but it must be designed to encourage the client to act. Please do not blindly take a national news release and send it to your clients. Don't try to give all the reasons for them to act. What is more important is that headings and subheadings are in order so when the brochure is skimmed the message still comes across in sequence. Any way the brochure is read, the reader needs to get the whole practice story and a feeling of the value-added benefits.

A recent development that has become an effective way to reach many of the female clients is the use of short quotes from famous literature. The quote selected should further illustrate the heading, accent a photo, or provide the reason that the client needs to keep reading and react. While the choice of literature says something about the quality and caring within the practice, so does adequate research to ensure the correct message is being sent.

Try to define your practice philosophy and scope of services in terms you believe will attract the type of clients you want to serve. They don't want to read about the practice philosophy; they want to experience it! Use bullets to highlight the three to six reasons that your practice is special. Put the proof of each claim in the center of white space so it will stand alone.

If you can do all this while giving the impression that your practice reduces the financial risk to the client, the copy will sell the practice to the uninformed but concerned pet owners.

Photos and Graphics

Copy is essential to the message, but graphics and photos can deliver the message faster and more effectively. Photos need to show activity and smiling and caring people and should indicate that healthcare will be successful. In some communities, people judge quality by the appearance of the staff, others by the appearance of the veterinarian or facility. Ensure that every photo sells the caring and confidence of the practice, rather than just sharing information about the appearance of the practice. As stated earlier, never print a photo when the size of the head is smaller than a dime. The graphics need to reinforce the main message and show what you want your target market to look like, both the clients (age, ethnicity, life style, etc.) and patients (canine, feline, avian, etc.).

The layout, the design, and even the type style (font) will add to the presentation of the graphics. Be very careful of colors in today's marketplace; brown-on-brown was good in the 1960s, the 1970s used a lot of maroon and grey, and in the 1980s orange and mauve were popular. It is important that you consult local design experts about what colors will be perceived as contemporary and appropriate.

As critical as colors is balance. A small animal hospital that only pictures dogs sends the message that cats are unimportant. If birds are not pictured and discussed, they will not appear in the exam room except by rare occurrence. Look at the dentistry photos around your practice; how many depict cats being treated?

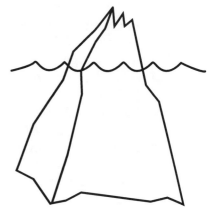

The graphics for the logo must be unique. Some have used footprints, some have used silhouettes, and others have used their own innovation to develop a logo that hasn't been seen in their community before. The consistency of use is important, but so is the practice identification (the veterinary symbol does not reflect any specific practice, just the profession). In certain community situations, an architectural sketch of the facility is the most effective logo. This logo, like a picture of the veterinarian, is unique and won't be duplicated by other practices.

Cost

How much should a brochure cost to produce? It depends on the talents of your staff, family, and friends. They understand what catches their attention in commercials, *USA Today,* or fliers that come to their homes; these people are not out for your money, nor do they have the glitter bias of a slick advertising executive. The need for a graphic design expert to develop a logo can often be filled by consulting a commercial artist or even a college's art department. Though not as innovative, the printer often costs less and can be very helpful about type and paper styles.

Most practices do not seek adequate resources to develop a brochure tailored to their practice philosophy *and* the community standards of quality in pet healthcare. Use all the resources available and do not rush into print; take the time to develop a brochure that will keep clients coming into the practice.

Implementation

There are many effective ways to use a practice brochure. Needless to say, new clients need to get one as they check in. Another method is to use it in response to a phone inquiry about the practice or prices; asking for an address may eliminate calls by competitors and will add value to your message for clients who really care. Most practices don't want to take the time or pay the cost of mailing a practice brochure to potential clients (sounds dumb, doesn't it?), so it is a method of differentiating a practice from others in most communities. My personal favorite is to include the brochure with the "thank you for referring someone to our practice" letter and tell the client I have included another brochure for the next friend he or she wants to refer.

The brochure is an excellent "leave behind" when a practice member speaks to any group in the community, including the schools since most all kids have parents, homes, and pets. Brochures can also be provided at county fairs, school awareness days, or health fairs presented by local hospitals. The leave behind benefit is also gained when you contact local media representatives to offer your practice as a resource when they need a veterinary healthcare perspective on some issue.

As a direct mail (cold call) piece, practice brochures seldom get the effect that is desired. There is seldom any cost-to-benefit advantage, since cost-effective direct mail needs to be less than 50¢ per piece including the mailing and development; good brochures usually cost more than this without mailing expenses. The good brochure is written for people who have already selected the practice (phone shoppers selected the practice—they just need help with selecting when to visit); the brochure should give them reasons to stay bonded to the practice. This is why a practice brochure is often an effective "leave behind" after a successful presentation; the audience has started bonding to the ideas of the speaker and thus to the practice.

Every quality practice needs a brochure to reinforce its position in the veterinary healthcare marketplace. It needs to be well developed, by local community people informed about *sales literature,* then molded to fit the philosophy of the practice. Those high-powered advertising folks in California will usually address an audience different from the conservative rancher, midwestern suburbanite, northeastern traditionalist, or southern good old friend of the practice. No one knows a practice's clients better than the staff, but most veterinarians cannot write good copy or develop a high-impact brochure. Use the resources within the staff to brainstorm with a local copywriter and graphic designer but keep control of the presentation and direction. Regardless of the community and practice philosophy, remember the basic rule in any healthcare marketing effort:

The only thing you really sell in healthcare is peace of mind. The client must be allowed to buy the services or products.

How to Use Newsletters Strategically

"Newsletters are a waste of time and money!" I have heard this statement at more practices than I wish to remember. It seems that if we mail a newsletter, new clients are supposed to line up at the door and demand admittance, slowed only by the hordes of returning clients who want to spend their money at our front counter. Newsletters seldom serve a significant role as stand-alone marketing efforts, but there is a place for well-written newsletters in practices that have a marketing plan or in practices that are concerned with reinforcing their clients' bond.

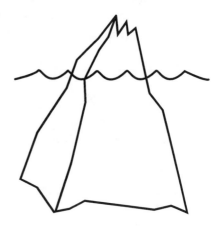

Frequency

Frequency of mailing is not dependent upon the newsletter but, rather, the marketing or business plans of the practice. A quarterly newsletter is just as ineffective as a bimonthly or semiannual unless you have targeted a desired marketing result. To cause front door traffic during the three slower seasons of the year, most proactive marketing plans require at least three newsletters. If your practice never has a slow season, you probably don't need a newsletter—you are already doing something right. In management as in practice, if it ain't broke, don't try to fix it.

If all seasons are slow, look to the bimonthly newsletter *after* you assess the real reason for the lack of clients. As previously stated, the business and marketing plans need to come first. They ensure marketing tools will be used in a selective and targeted manner.

Client Bonding

Client bonding is simply the desire of a client to drive by other clinics in favor of yours. The more facilities a client drives by, the better the client bond. In the modern urban marketplace, it can also be measured by monitoring the number of new clients referred each month by your existing clients. We usually expect about 40 new clients per veterinarian per month in a mature practice; if we believe the Charles, Charles, and Associates 1988 report to the American Veterinary Medical Association, we'd expect about 60 percent of new clients to come by way of personal referral in a highly bonded client base.

An item of interest that Catanzaro & Associates has noticed visiting about 800 veterinary facilities a year is that the store-bought newsletters are less effective than those tailored to the locality and practice. In fact, some of the best newsletters feature a different staff member in each issue, profiling him or her as a real person that lives in the community. Another effective newsletter method includes discussing issues of interest to the community, such as parasite populations in flooding or drought. This approach makes veterinary concern much more real for the readers.

Marketing Methods

The newsletter can become an important part of a marketing plan. If the newsletter targets a special interest and is followed by a cause for action, the combination can be magnificent.

◆ EXAMPLE 1: In early November, a newsletter mailed to current clients discusses the dangers of overweight lifestyles to pets. This is the season when most clients notice their own weight gain, so that is an added advantage. A newsletter sidebar can discuss dental problems, holiday food dangers, how quality wellness care affects nutrition and health, as well as the reduction of mouth odors with regular dentistries. Now comes the follow-up that makes the difference.

• Option A—Send a postcard in early January announcing free counseling by the practice's nutritional counselors (technicians or receptionists that have completed a criteria-based training program).

• Option B—If you are computerized, send a January postcard to all households that have had pets show a weight gain in the previous year and remind them that inactivity in the winter months increases the chances for weight gain. Offer them an opportunity to have a free predental exam when they bring their pet in for nutritional counseling.

• Option C—Send a January postcard to owners of all pets that had a two-plus mouth (grading system based on pictures, as discussed in Vol. 2, *Building the Successful Veterinary Practice*) and were not enrolled in a dental program. Remind clients that now is the time for a follow-up exam to ensure that the problem hasn't gotten worse and that proper nutritional standards are being maintained so that their pets can live longer, healthier lives.

• Option D—Combine two of the above—be innovative and creative!

◆ EXAMPLE 2: In early February, a Valentine's Day newsletter is sent to all dog owners. It highlights the current status of heartworms in your locality and the availability of Heartguard as a once per month program (or Interceptor in a heavy parasite area). A sidebar can be added discussing ECG capabilities of the practice, the special short courses you and your staff have recently attended, and geriatric concerns in an annual heart checkup.

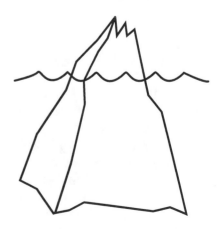

• Option A—Send a postcard in late February announcing a special heartworm screening clinic in the evenings to reduce scheduling hassles for busy families.

• Option B—Send a postcard in early March announcing a special geriatric physical program, with an ECG, that also includes a free predental examination or free nutritional assessment.

• Option C—Use your computer to target all pets that have not had a refill for their heartworm preventive and/or to target all pets that have been annotated as geriatric during their most recent visits. Impart this information in a postcard.

• Option D—Ask the staff for a new twist to the above options, such as "P.S. Our spring two-fur-one special is bring in a stool sample from two of your pets and we will examine them for the price of one—family health is important to us!"

◆ EXAMPLE 3: You don't publish a newsletter because you are exactly where you want to be in your practice growth, and the status quo is comfortable.

• Option A—Remember, the CPI has been over 4 percent each year and an additional 6 percent plus is needed for your retirement. Are you ready?

• Option B—In medicine, stasis is associated with death; in practice management, it is not much different.

• Option C—The choice does belong to the hospital director, as does the practice success.

• Option D—Reassess the entire practice situation, from staff as well as client perspectives. Is it time for succession planning.

Writing the Newsletter

The most important thing to remember in writing a newsletter is the audience you want to continue to attract (yes folks, "continue to attract"; writing a newsletter is a bond-maintaining device). One of the best resources in your quest for the best newsletter composition is the staff. They hear what the clients are concerned about. Use this resource.

In the development of the newsletter, ensure some, if not all, of the content is tailored to your specific community and practice. The generic and nationally sold newsletters make money for those that sell them, but generally those profits are not shared by the users. The other thing to use is the current media literature on hot pet owner issues.

A New Client newsletter (Fig. 3.3), something that shares more than the pictures in the brochure, should be left on the front counter for long periods of time and should be sent to *every* phone shopper.

The two-column format in Figure 3.3 makes the practice's message look more like a newsletter, although it's not a requirement. The graphics used are minimal, since one picture really is worth a thousand words. Consider using a behind-the-scenes picture, which clients love. The layout and content must be tailored to the practice; colors must be consistent among issues; messages from the doctors, staff, and newsletter must be compatible.

It is interesting to note that the sample newsletter in Figure 3.3 can be printed on an 11×17-inch page (in a color that matches your stationary color), which can be folded to make a real four-page newsletter (which explains the weird page numbering). Like the brochure, the new client newsletter is designed to inform the potential clients of how the practice is different from others, why they need to try the services, and why they can have confidence in the quality of the care being offered.

The emphasis in human healthcare has shifted from just curing illness to maintaining and restoring wellness. The media are covering this trend, and clients are beginning to expect this approach in veterinary healthcare. To do so, a practice needs to enter into a partnership with a concerned pet owner. It must tell the client what is needed and educate him or her as to the consequences if the care is not accessed. Quite often, a *health alert* can precede a specific program. The health alert is an informative newsletter about a single subject, as illustrated in Figure 3.4. A health alert newsletter can have greater impact if the borders and title are red. A bulk run of stock paper can be preprinted and used in a photocopier to produce the newsletters for a target mailing.

Newsletters and health alerts should promote the practice's team effort to restore wellness. Some practices even endorse their referral practice colleagues in these media and mention that patients will be referred to specialists when other expertise is needed, whether it be an emergency clinic, a university, or a Board-certified specialist. Pictures of the healthcare delivery team members can be featured in a new client newsletter (heads the size of a dime or larger, never smaller), with pictures on the wall (with titles and hopefully their pets), or in the clinic brochure (generally as a supplemental insert). The team does include the paraprofessional staff, and they need to be recognized for their contribution.

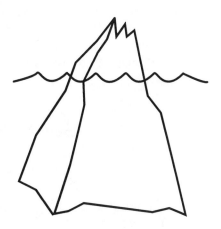

If you want to convey quality in newsletters, do not shortcut the development process. The client newsletter can be ben-

SPECIAL PROGRAMS AT ACME CLINIC	WELCOME & "HOWDY" NEWSLETTER
Concerned Pet Owners................................ .... ask about our PREFERRED CLIENT PROGRAM........ .... ☺ ☺ ☺ ☺ ☺ .... Plan A is the............................. Health Maintenance .... available for puppies and kittens, adult pets, and our senior friends.. We offer advantages to .... to clients that prepay.. ....for a wellness "bundle" .... of pet care........... Dental................. ..with puppy or kitten ....vaccination bundles, ...we also provide a fecal sample examination for dangerous internal parasites as an added benefit .... ☺ ☺ ☺ ☺ ☺ .... Golden Years Program....................... .... Cancer Rider to the DVM/VPI National Catastrophic Pet Health Insurance .... Plan B .... ☺ ☺ ☺ ☺ ☺ Our RESPITE BOARDING PROGRAM is reserved for our patients with medical conditions requiring skilled professional care during the absence of their stewards 4	ACME VETERINARY CLINIC WELCOMES YOU & YOUR PET Dr. __ Dr. -- Ms. ?? Mr. ?? owner associate Hosp mgr Resort Mgr Dr. ___ has been in the community............................ enjoys .... and .... Dr. _____ joined our team in 19__ and originally hails from ....she has been active in................................. has a special interest in .... enjoys .... Ms. xxx, our lead nurse technician.......................is a native of .... prefers to maintain and restore wellness rather than just cure illness .... is active in the .... Ms. Judy ?? became our hospital manager .... has trained _____ staff, and is the most requested person on our phones. Mr. *** has been our lead receptionist since .... and .... has two cats, Merlin and Sabbath, a major sized white Alaskan Malamute named Tara, a tenured pigmy goat who sometimes answers to Farley, and a small herd of .... Mr. _____ is our resort manager and our behavior specialist, ... new pet owner classes... .... puppy and kitten classes ....

Fig. 3.3. Format for new client newsletter.

eficial to your practice, but a strategic plan will be required. Use your staff to develop the plan; then empower your team to implement it and monitor success. Have them feel they can unilaterally make changes to better reach clients and meet their pets' needs. Publishing a newsletter needs a team effort.

Service Is an Obligation

An appointment is a contract and must be kept—on time!

During the past decade, the average work week decreased from about 80 hours to 55 hours for most veterinarians. Yet the majority of practicing veterinarians continually report they do not have enough leisure time.

OTHER HEALTHCARE THOUGHTS	SAMPLE PROGRAMS
ACME Veterinary clinic .... believes in involving each client in the treatment plan for their pet .... ☺ ☺ ☺ ☺ ☺ We need a partnership with you.................................. properly react when the .... we need to enter a baseline of wellness .... next illness occurs................................ We will tell you what needs to be done .... you will be part of our healthcare delivery team .... for the best care, but you must tell us what you want done ....to better assist you .... when not available, we will ask you to use our Emergency Service ....which we trust and respect, working with their specialists .... ☺ ☺ ☺ ☺ ☺ ☺ For our established clients, we offer a comprehensive nursing counselor program as an additional courtesy, but scheduled for your time benefit, including .... to discuss parasite control.................. ....fleas.............ticks..............heartworms............ ....even internal worms which can be transmitted to children...............................nutrition .... and dental concerns like bad breath and .... ☺ ☺ ☺ ☺ ☺ ☺	Any abdominal surgery requires an "exclusive use", aseptic surgery suite, ...pre-surgical lab .... post-surgical care .... post-anesthetic pain killers .... trained recovery staff .... clear discharge instructions... the American College of Veterinary Anesthesiologists has stated .... that every pet undergoing general anesthesiology deserves .... certain levels of laboratory assessment... ....post care.. ☺ ☺ ☺ ☺ ☺ An ovariohysterectomy is a major abdominal surgery, not just a .... "spay".. .... pre-care includes .... An orchectomy (castration) .... also requires aseptic techniques.. post care................. and.. ☺ ☺ ☺ ☺ ☺ Oral hygiene is important in animals .... ☺ ☺ ☺ ☺ ☺ Arthritis surveillance.. .... ☺ ☺ ☺ ☺ ☺ Cardiac evaluations and other essential "over 40" medical checks start at about 6 years of age in most companion animals and include............................... ....
We also offer you our nurse technician HOT LINE to help answer those little or passing questions that all pet owners have from time to time .... nutrition .... poison ....coughing ....limping ....6 a.m. to 8 p.m.	
2	3

Fig. 3.3. (*continued*)

Many practitioners open earlier, stay later, and have expanded to weekend appointment hours. The six-day work week is *still* the norm. There is legislation pending in some states to address the staffing of veterinary facilities after-hours. This is a financial challenge to the future of our profession.

Veterinarians are a caring lot and go out of their way to tend to the needs of their clients and patients. That is why we entered the profession. I don't know of anyone who entered it primarily to become a millionaire. The expanding clinical hours in the veterinary practice community have been a response to public demand as well as a method to increase income. With most urban and suburban families headed by dual-wage earners or single parents, evening and weekend convenience is needed. When located in a metroplex, a practice of-

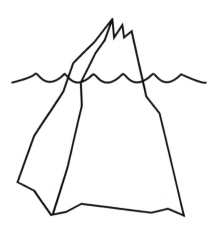

VETERINARY MEDICAL HEALTH ALERT
Courtesy of Acme Veterinary Clinic

DATELINE:

Large Type Headline (single issue)

Discovery statement on the most alarming or attention getting aspect of the new health issue being shared ....

Zoonotic threat to the family, pet owner, or threat to other animals ....

Research basis or incidence rate within the specific community of the veterinary health alert distribution........ ....

Preventative measures that are now available ....

Wellness concerns for pets and other animals they may come into contact with ....

What to do if there is a suspected case, ... home care.. ....versus ....when to see their veterinarian ....

CONCERNED or WORRIED?
FOR ADDITIONAL INFORMATION,
PLEASE CALL:

Fig. 3.4. Sample health alert newsletter.

fering a morning drop-off is filling a market niche based on service.

The use of an appointment system is still evolving. The walk-in system generally gave way to 15–30 minute appointments a decade ago, and the 20-minute appointment became commonplace by the end of the 1980s. Now the flexible 10-minute appointment log has been introduced to allow tailoring of the practice's appointment times. There are still a few walk-in practices, and some appointment-only practices have adopted a friendlier stance for walk-ins by using their inpatient teams to handle them.

Ten-minute flexible scheduling works like this: 10 minutes for recheck or suture removal, 20 minutes for outpatient sick call, an extra 10 minutes for new clients to discuss practice philosophy, an extra 10 minutes for a second or third animal, an extra 10 minutes to discuss husbandry for an exotic patient, an extra 10 minutes for a senior citizen benefit in lieu of a discount, or the extra 10 minutes needed for a new graduate to do anything. Using these general guidelines to develop the practice's appointment program is essential, but the real secret lies in high-density scheduling for the doctor.

In *high-density scheduling,* the doctor and outpatient nurse work as a team. They have two examination rooms, and no one is allowed to divert the nurse from supporting the doctor in these two rooms. High-density scheduling is based on overlapping the last 10 minutes of one appointment in one room with the first 10 minutes of the next appointment in the other room. The staggered schedule just means the outpatient nurse loads the other room and does the 3 to 5 minute wellness screen 10 minutes before the end of the preceding appointment, puts the record with findings on a rack outside the rear door of the exam room, and then returns to the room with the doctor. When the nurse enters, the doctor knows it is time to immediately disengage and transfer client education and closeout to the nurse. Then the doctor moves to the other room, reviewing the wellness screen recorded in the medical record by the outpatient nurse, who left it on the rear door of the examination room. Veterinary medicine is the only healthcare profession where the primary provider works in a linear fashion, which I attribute to the "farm call, pickup truck, one-at-a-time, do it yourself practice foundation" of those who went before. The companion animal practice facility was first established in 1938, and that makes most of the people we learned from mixed animal practitioners. The results of entering the high-density scheduling world include

- Fifty percent more client care in a shorter period of time.
- In fact, once the doctor and nurse have worked out the bugs, a full day's workload is generally done in a half-day schedule (16 to 18 patients).
- Morning outpatient teams become afternoon inpatient teams, increasing their productivity. They finish their day admissions and do the discharges on morning surgery cases.
- The gross income is therefore increased accordingly, but the gross expenses do not spiral up at the same rate, so the practice sees increased net.

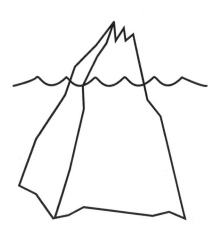

Marketing Advantages of Scheduling

In Yellow Pages advertising and media marketing, quality practices center on service to differentiate their facilities from others. They use phrases like "evening hours," "walk-ins welcomed any time," "Visa, MC, American Express, and Discover accepted," "weekend hours." This is very effective for the well-informed or well-bonded clients, but the less-bonded and poorly informed clients still pursued cost savings with vigor. Interestingly, the lower-end (discount-type) practices have been most susceptible to failure during the recent recession. For the first time in history, the 1990s saw veterinary practices closing in response to hard times (reportedly at a 10 percent rate in cities like Toronto, Colorado Springs, and Oregon).

Saturday hours are still the most popular, but the pressures of Saturday are being shifted to newly offered hours: Sunday hours and 5:00 to 8:00 p.m. weekdays. While this is not all bad, the tendency during these hectic appointment times is to just treat the problem and not the patient. The need for return visits is overlooked, the more intensive diagnostics are waived or deferred, and some concurrent or underlying problems are never addressed. Shifting away from quality veterinary healthcare costs the practice net income, even if increasing volume increases the gross.

There are companion animal practices with appointment hours only from noon to 8:00 p.m. They support a bedroom community of commuters. There are practices that have morning appointments until 10:00 a.m. and do not schedule appointments again until after 3:00 p.m.; surgery is a midday activity, as are mobile home calls. New companion animal veterinary facilities are being built with an odd number of exam rooms so the doctor-nurse pairs can work two rooms and the odd room can be used by the in-patient team to see walk-ins and emergencies in a timely manner, without disrupting the high-density scheduling.

Compounding these scheduling problems has been the inherent fear of client fee resistance, usually unfounded in an established practice (except for quotables). As a rule, during the first years of the 1990s, veterinary practices found their gross slightly increase but their net decrease. The client's ability and willingness to pay for services have been put to the test: practices have raised their fees, and the average transaction charge has been going upward. But client demand for veterinary service has not fallen off. The smarter practices have developed discharge planning programs that increase the client return rate rather than the average transaction fee. More smaller ticket visits over a period of time support the client perception that the practices have lower costs.

The greatest impetus for extended hours is competition from other practices. Colleges of veterinary medicine in the United States and Canada have increased the number of graduates during the 1990s, and almost every animal owner now has multiple veterinarians to select from. For this reason, the fear of competition is founded. If you close Saturday, your clients will find a different practice. If you take a vacation without a relief veterinarian, clients will go elsewhere, some never to return. In communities without competition, Saturday hours are less important. If you are the only game in town, you set the table rules!

To get a multiveterinarian practice into a quality of life program, Catanzaro & Associates uses a basic prototype of a two-week scheduling cycle for the professional staff. The sequence is two days on, one off, three days on, one off, four days on, then a three-day weekend. The second veterinarian starts the same schedule, but a week later. In a two-doctor practice, this single staffs the practice on Friday-Saturday-Sunday, but double staffs it on Monday, Tuesday, and Thursday (Wednesday is church night in many communities, so we recommend not fighting it). High-density scheduling increases the number of clients seen. The double-staffing days allow for evening hours because one veterinarian can come in later (e.g., 1:00 p.m.) and work until 7:00 or 8:00 p.m. with evening appointment hours.

As the profession expands, the need to cooperate with our colleagues will outweigh the need to compete. Be the first in your area to generate professional conversation concerning meeting the community's needs through rotating office hours. Meeting the needs of clients while meeting the needs of your staff and self will become increasingly important.

Communicating to Win

The man who will use his skill and constructive imagination to see how much he can give for a dollar, instead of how little he can give for a dollar, is bound to succeed.
—Henry Ford

PetsMart, Wal-Mart, even the grocery store down the street are competing for the pet healthcare dollar. Some large format retailers even hire corporations that provide low-cost veterinarians. What this competition does not have is a technician-veterinarian healthcare delivery team. The veterinarian may produce the gross income, but the technician can produce the net income required for survival and prosperity. In a progressive veterinary practice, together you offer a caring and trusted alternative to concerned pet owners.

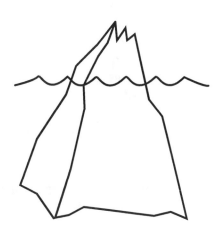

The worse the news, the more effort should go into communicating it.
                                    —*A. S. Grove*

Communication is simply the getting and giving of information. When consumers enter a discount store, they expect less quality and better prices and look forward to finding a bargain. The communication that occurs is usually price centered. When consumers enter a healthcare facility, even if they are stressed, they still expect a fair price, but they expect quality as well. There is an unspoken social contract:

1. First, the facility will do no harm.

2. Second, the providers will only do what is needed.

3. Third, there will be a fair fee assessed for the services rendered.

4. Fourth, all parties want to restore wellness in the patient.

In the examination room, most veterinarians use technical terms, which would be appropriate if this jargon was explained; however, it seldom is. Most clients don't know about the most common terms, like FVRCP, DHLAPP, FeLV, or FIV, and understand less about the -itis, -osis, -ectomy, and even "benign" findings. (A recent survey by the American College of Healthcare Executives showed 46 percent of the population did not understand the term "benign" when used with "cancer.")

Clients deserve to be told what is needed, and why. They deserve the opportunity to ask questions. They deserve the respect of the healthcare provider. When these steps have been taken, clients need to be asked for their position. The phrase may be "What seems fair for your pet today?" or "Do you want us to start today, or would you like to make an appointment for a return visit?" or some other request that will elicit a positive reply. Do not advocate levels of care, just alternative options that require a yes response. When a "maybe," a stall, or a question is the reply, then react in accordance with the situation. Regardless of the reply, client bonding requires that you take the 30 to 60 seconds needed to validate their decisions. This short effort gets them back through the door. This is positive communication.

Speech is a mirror of the soul; as a man speaks, so he is.
                                    —*Publilius Syrus*

Your first response to the suggestion that you allow time to communicate with clients may be "There isn't enough time in the day!" Does that mean you don't want clients to come back, or does it mean you don't want clients to be supportive of the treatment plan offered? There are alternatives to the doctor being responsible for all the examination room communication. In most veterinary practices in America, there exists at least one underutilized staff member waiting to be developed. Doctors try to do too much themselves and, in turn, don't do enough for each client and pet. Ask yourself these questions about your practice's pet health counseling system:

Who does the nutritional counseling?
- Are serial weights in every medical record?
- Who does the monthly client recall, patient appearance recheck, and weigh-ins?
- Who monitors the client's reorder point for prescription diets?
- Who discusses the home supplementation concerns when the client stops the prescription diet feeding?

Who does the parasite prevention and control counseling?
- Does the practice understand the difference between foggers and a premises eradication guarantee (such as Fleabusters)?
- Who actually defines where in the house (floor plan assessments) foggers need to go for most effect versus a total premises plan?
- Who does the follow-up to ensure there was effective elimination?
- Who ensures the external parasite and internal parasite relationships (e.g., tapeworms, anemia, etc.) are understood by the client?

Who does the dental hygiene counseling?
- Are clients allowed to go home and are they asked to rub the pet's teeth nightly with tuna water (cats) or garlic water (dogs) before they come back and discuss dental options? Who does this return visit counseling?
- Who takes the time to discuss the diet and bad breath effects of poor teeth?
- Who cares enough to tell clients that "red gums mean pain" and to explain the healthcare options?

Who does the behavior management counseling?
- Does it automatically start with the puppy/kitten series?
- Is house-training assistance given during the first puppy/kitten visit as a value-added service?
- Who spends time listening to the

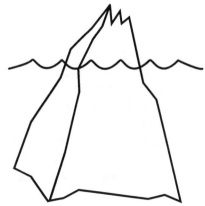

client's needs? (Eighty-five percent of clients report that they do have a pet behavior problem.)
- Who schedules short familiarization times in the clinic, on a weekly basis, to help change the unwanted behavior?
- Who does the callbacks to ensure the behavior management ideas are being implemented in the home, with all the family members participating?

Who does the client callbacks?
- Are new clients called and told, "Welcome to our practice"?
- Are postmedication-dispensing calls made (halfway through treatment) to ensure clients do not have questions (and haven't stopped the treatment program or forgotten the recheck appointment)?
- Are postsurgical calls made, at recovery and again four days after discharge, to ensure the client has no worries?
- Who does discharge planning follow-up (form is in Vol. 2, Appendix C)?

These are just a few situations where the receptionist-technician team members can extend the effectiveness of the veterinarian. Veterinary extenders may also be reminder postcards, established staff protocols, laboratory result telephone calls to the client, or a host of other client service-oriented activities. Clients should perceive a higher level of service and caring at a veterinary hospital (the pet health expert in the community) than they do at discount pet stores, and in most practices, 80 percent of clients' contact has traditionally been with the paraprofessional staff. It is the caring and knowledge of the technician and receptionist that allow the client to form that favorable first impression of the practice image.

The Patient Advocate

Man is a dog's ideal of what God should be.

—Holbrook Jackson

It is the responsibility of the veterinary healthcare team to speak for the needs of the animals they care for—to be their advocates. Concurrently, we must give clients the right to make informed decisions, which means we should take the time to explain an animal's needs and, on many occasions, the alternatives available to meet those needs. The greater the clients' knowledge of the healthcare needs (their veterinary I.Q.), the more often their pets will receive the needed care.

The patient advocate desires the best care possible, but the clients' budgets determine what they can afford, which may be only part of what is needed during any given pay period (proof of this is your paycheck each pay period). It is the paraprofessional healthcare provider who can keep in touch with clients and get them to return the following month for some of the other care needed. The enthusiasm and caring of the technician or receptionist can help make this return decision a practice reality. When a staff member becomes a healthcare team member, client communications improve. Many clients feel more comfortable discussing concerns with the technician because (1) they don't want to take the doctor's time, (2) they don't understand the terms the veterinarian uses, or, simply, (3) they feel it is easier to talk to the technician or the receptionist. The clients' concerns must be addressed if the practice wants the clients to return, and these concerns are first told to a staff member, not the doctor. This is why the staff member has such a great influence on the number of clients entering a practice.

The technician team needs to work with the receptionist team to ensure that narratives are understood and clients are knowledgeable about every practice program and service. When a client calls about a flea or tick problem, does the client sense the urgency, if any, associated with treating this problem? Can the fleas and ticks be handled with a bath and some dusting powder from a pet store? What level of in-service education about fleas and ticks has been conducted for the staff members at your hospital? Do they know about the other diseases that are often screened for in a tick or flea case (e.g., Lyme disease, tapeworms, etc.) and how to best communicate this need to clients? Some veterinary practices have initiated a technician hotline just to ensure the client can reach someone who has the time to care. What client education skills has your practice developed in staff members who talk to clients on the phone, at the front desk, or in the exam room? How are they reinforced? Who is the patient advocate?

Steps for Communicating to Win

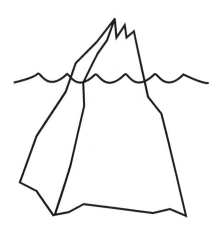

It takes two to speak the truth—one to speak and one to hear.
—Henry David Thoreau

Most clients are not well-informed consumers of veterinary healthcare services. They do not understand how much the levels of quality and training vary among suppliers. Our profession hasn't helped this situation too much. We still deal in "quotables" on a daily basis. Communicating to win is not selling a service or product. It is letting people buy.

If we assume listening to clients is a given (which it seldom is unless we train ourselves to do so), then we meet their needs and wants *first*. In veterinary healthcare delivery, we often discover additional needs of the patient during the physical examination; these must be prioritized into the care plan. Communicating to win has four basic steps that any practice can learn to follow:

1. Make the client aware of a *pre-existing* condition that needs attention.

2. Educate the client about the changes in the veterinary profession that now allow you to address the condition.

3. With caring and enthusiasm, offer your practice's program to address the client's concern (the patient's problem).

4. After the client replies, validate the response, regardless of what it is, and set the expectation for the next encounter.

Veterinary clients base most decisions on the emotion of the moment, while the average veterinary practice addresses the logic of the need. Logic will seldom answer the emotional need, but staff members who care can. The pet owner wants to know how much you care, not how much you know. Clients expect professional excellence when they contact a veterinarian's office, so don't disappoint them by recommending a "tincture of time" brush-off. They also want caring, so never disappoint them in this area either!

The opening contact with a client should be nonthreatening (avoid questions that require only a yes or no answer) and should be used to gather information. Phone shoppers should be mailed a hospital brochure, newsletter, or flyer the same day they call, so their addresses must be recorded. They need to know that the practice treats the whole animal and cares for the whole family. When healthcare recommendations are made, they need to be stated as "needs." Be clear about the needs of the animal or of the practice. For instance, a preanesthesia laboratory profile is a professional need to ensure there isn't something going on that cannot be seen that may cause anesthetic complications. Explain the entire wellness approach of the practice, for animals as well as their owners.

After the low-key conversational greeting, the information gathering, and the valuation of total wellness, the client must make the decision to buy. As already mentioned, if the smart technician or receptionist offers two alternatives, both of which require a yes response, the ability to buy is assisted. The best way for someone to "close a sale" varies with the service, the product, and the individuals involved in the discussion. But regardless of the closure method, one additional step is needed. A caring practice must ensure it makes the client comfortable about his or her decision. Whether the client opts for full service, partial care, deferred service, or simply waiving the care, you want him or her to return to the practice another time. Return visits make a greater net for the practice than the search for new clients, so discussing a client's next visit is part of the "comforting" action. If the dental decision was "not today ... ," assign a technician to make a telephone follow-up to establish the expectation for a return visit. You accept them and their decisions, but you want to see them again!

> *Glory is fleeting, but obscurity is forever.*
> —*Napoleon Bonaparte*

These ideas for improving communication do not guarantee success; they only allow you to add to the practice's success. How you empower the staff to extend veterinary caring will make a difference. But how you deliver this caring will make the real difference. Follow Star Trek Captain Jean-Luc Picard's approach and make it so!

Council of Clients

> *If you want to better know how to serve your clients, ask them!*
> —*Dr. T. E. Cat*

The average veterinary practitioner is so knowledgeable, he or she knows what the client wants without even asking them—right? Wrong. Satisfaction is only a passing perception of our clients, and to promote this we must capture their opinions.

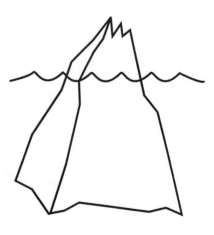

Bring Them Together

The Council of Clients is simply a dozen or so clients, with their spouses or significant others, who join you for dessert one evening during the quarter. The council, formed for one meeting, focuses on what needs to be done to better support the community and clients of your practice. The group configuration can be varied each quarter: clients with highest tickets, those with most visits, third-reminder phone contacts, home owner association members, breeders, cat owners, or whatever special interest or classification you desire. The idea is to get new ideas. If you're well versed in survey techniques, this is basically a tailored focus group.

Key Elements for Success

What to say to yourself before the meeting

"My clients know what they want to buy; I need to meet that need. I believe in getting feedback from my clients; I will go out of my comfort zone to get it. Their opinions make my job easier and keep the practice going strong."

Focus group questions

Determine the purpose of bringing a focus group together, specifically for this meeting as well as for practice use after the meeting.

Example: "The purpose of this meeting is to get a general consensus of how we are doing in servicing our client needs." (Overview)

Example: "The purpose of this meeting is to explore new ways to serve you and the community." (More specific)

The focus group composition and opening questions will depend on the purpose of the meeting. After deciding on the purpose, develop a group of questions to drive the discussions.

Introduction to participants

Set the tone and expectations.

1. "We want to make sure our hospital is satisfying your needs and expectations."

2. "We appreciate your being here this evening and appreciate your feedback."

3. State the purpose of the meeting.

Brainstorming Procedures

The purpose of any client meeting is to get a lot of ideas to enhance practice services.

1. List all ideas offered by group members on easel paper and hang completed sheets on the wall for continuous viewing.

2. Do not evaluate or judge ideas at this time.

3. Do not discuss ideas, except perhaps briefly, to clarify understanding.

4. Welcome any idea. It is always easier to eliminate than to accumulate.

5. Encourage quantity. The more ideas, the greater the likelihood of a useful one.

Stimulating discussion
Overview question:

1. "Could you tell me two or three things you like about our hospital?"

2. "Could you identify the one thing we need to do to improve our service?"

Specific survey questions:

1. "If we were to offer the following three services, which would be most beneficial to your pet and your family?"

2. "How could we keep you better informed of the status of the treatment we are providing your pet?"

3. "What can we do to better communicate the needs of your pet and our desire to serve you?"

Provide feedback to the participants

1. Recognize their ideas as caring with "I haven't looked at it that way," "That is a unique perspective we haven't researched yet," or even responses like "Great!", "Thank you!", "Right on," "That is a winner!" or other positive replies.

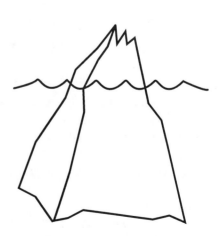

2. If participants suggest services you already offer, don't tell them. Say, "The (ideas) will be in effect by the first of next week—thank you!"

3. When you put a transition or marketing plan together to implement the ideas in an organized manner, send the participants a copy *so they know what action has been taken on their recommendations.*

Bang for the Buck

Do not ask a question if you are not ready to hear the response. Do not ask high-ticket clients to participate in a Council of Clients if you don't want to talk about cost of care. If you invite seniors, get ready for AARP questions, including senior discounts and larger print handouts. The Council of Clients is not just an exercise in feeding some of the community a dessert once a quarter. It is meant to give the practice information needed to make rapid and targeted changes for the good of the business and the clients it supports.

Do not define perceptions out of existence, they are real to those who hold them. For example a spouse or significant other will give a second-hand impression of what went on with a patient visit. This may point out the need for improved handouts. To benefit from the Council of Clients, be prepared to listen. Listen to what participants mean as well as what they say. These are not always the same. Listen to the perceived trends and the feelings of the clients. Capitalize on this encounter by making the practice respond to their needs. Offer more services, package them differently, or just offer them at different times or in different ways. "Bang for the buck" means that those who attended the Council of Clients feel as if they were heard and believe the practice wants to make things better for the community. Without these feelings and beliefs, a bang will occur, but probably without the buck.

Programs = Net Income

As I was surfing the Net, I watched veterinarians discuss their 1995 increase in gross, the percentage of gross that was due to vaccines or dentistry, and other such first-liar-loses discussions. When are we going to learn? *You can only take home the net!*

The Front Door Must Swing

Every practice has a different formula for making the front door swing, but there are common components called *programs* (as in program-based budgeting). For example, a preanesthetic laboratory screen should be done for virtually every surgery (although the intensity and scope will vary), and as stated in a recent Nevada State Board letter, 80 percent of the surgery cases should have fluids running. (When was the last time you took a fluid therapy refresher for continuing education [CE]?) Practices that record the grades of dental conditions in their medical records have used this information to step up their dental programs and double their incomes. One practice has even contacted Dr. Marv Samuelson for assistance in developing dermatology as an income center program (even in Colorado, 15 percent of the dogs coming in the front door have atopy).

There are many programs practices take for granted, especially in radiology. Fact: most every practice has forgotten that a radiographic baseline of the thorax is good medicine. A boarder who is coughing does not always have kennel cough. Dogs do have other problems. For instance, a negative Difil test gives you information about circulating microfilaria, not adult heartworms in the thorax. Only an X ray can do this effectively. Consider this: Dr. Bob Smith (radiologist, University of California, Davis) believes that dogs with a negative *or* positive heartworm test still deserve a thoracic X-ray series before starting the preventive care or treatment protocol. Moving on to the abdomen, when was the last time you did an IVP or cystogram? There are more things than just foreign bodies occurring in the abdomen. Have you ever considered the diagnostic advantage of a Barospheres when doing laparotomies, since leakage is not a by-product of these pellets? During a short course it was stated, "Use of the Penn Hip technique to aid in the diagnosis of hip dysplasia and the introduction of Baro-spheres for barium studies have proven diagnostic advantages." One client attending the course knew he could go back to his practice and virtually double his income in this area.

Economics

"Tom Cat, we will damage our relationship if we add unneeded diagnostics." You are right, if they are unneeded. But in every case stated above, there was a medical need. The fact that you have taken radiology for granted means the overhead is still larger than the income from the program center. Yes, program center—not income center, not profit center. The front door swings because you believe in your healthcare programs and share that conviction with clients. If you don't believe a diagnostic is medically needed, never do it!

And for those of you who take one film to

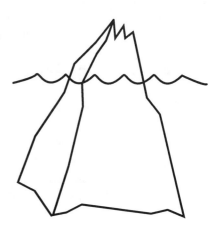

"save the client money," remember what every text and radiologist has stated, "If it looks like a duck, sounds like a duck, and walks like a duck, it must be considered a duck ... and ducks state very clearly, quack, quack, quack!" If radiology is needed, two views are needed. To provide half the care is a violation of professional ethics and the Practice Act. Think of a lameness case where you said, "If this does not get better, we may need to take radiographs." The client brought a suffering animal to you because she wanted peace of mind, and you only offered tincture of time. And you wonder why she didn't come back? Lameness generally requires radiology to determine the appropriate treatment as well as the prognosis; clients come to you because you are the diagnostician.

Belief in good medicine is the cornerstone of a successful practice. The ability to convey this need to clients is the cornerstone of a profitable practice. The overhead of a veterinary practice is pretty fixed (in well-managed practices, less than 50 percent of the gross income is spent on monthly expenses, not counting rent, doctor monies, and return on investment [ROI] benefits). So it is the delivery of services and products by existing staff, as well as facility capabilities, which can make the net income difference.

Today Is the First Day of the Rest of Your Life

We really don't care what you have already done. That is past. What we care about is what you are willing to do. Every year, new continuing education courses mean you have the opportunity to enhance practice programs. The continuing education experience that does not add one new program per day of CE attended is a wasted expense. A new program is designed to provide better care, and there is a value associated with that client benefit. That value, as assessed to clients, should be reflected in your program-based budget for the year. The cash flow reports from that computer in your office only reflect the belief level of the providers in the new programs being offered. When you believe in a program, the clients will accept the care as needed and essential. It is your choice—lower the net each year or provide better healthcare delivery programs. Just do it!

Bundling Services

When clients don't fall for prices, prices must fall for clients.

And the companion animal practitioner laments: "How can I compete with those spay and neuter humane societies/superstores/established practices/vaccination clinics/low-cost new graduates?" The voice from the wilderness says, "Meet their needs and they shall come." No client ever leaves a practice he or she is bonded to unless someone violates the social contract. This social contract is unwritten but clearly states, "For the money I pay you, I have peace of mind, and I received more veterinary healthcare than what I paid for during this encounter." One modality that can attract and retain the upper end clients (whose pets are family members) is the concept of bundled services.

Bundling veterinary healthcare services (promoting a multivisit service for a lower single cost) has become as common as specialty practices, but not all practices are ready for this concept. Clients are ready, since discretionary income has become tighter, but some practices have defined this factor out of existence. Bundling services means simply to take individual invoice items or procedures and combine them into a special program for the benefit of the client and pet. Some veterinary computer companies have developed invoice bundling as a template within their programs. Others will do it if you demand performance from their programmers.

Health Maintenance Agreements

Two of the most common health maintenance agreements (HMAs) are the puppy and kitten programs. In both, the entire preventive medicine program for the first four months is covered by a single price. This is the initial form of an HMA. Health maintenance agreements are basically self-insured pet wellness systems; they have been offered by certain practices for years. Some practices have even specialized their programs according to species and life cycle period: pediatric, adult, or geriatric. The standard healthcare elements have traditionally been composed of

1. Written physical examinations

2. A full vaccination series

3. Two fecal examinations

4. Annual heartworm/FeLV screening

5. Dental hygiene counseling (and two dental prophies in adults)

6. Two office calls, or "professional consultations"

7. Nutritional counseling

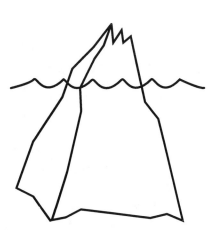

8. Parasite prevention and control assistance

9. Primary access to outpatient nurse assistance

Any form of emergency healthcare service is usually not included. However, for marketing purposes, this is also practice dependent. For instance, part of parasite prevention and control in the Southeast often includes two baths and dips, with one being done while the premises are treated (e.g., a Fleabusters program).

Each wellness program element in the HMA is clearly priced, with an individual value that is then mathematically bundled into an annual wellness program fee. The discounting is due strictly to a prepayment requirement. Blood chemistry or urinalysis screening has been included by some practices as value-added elements to differentiate their quality care programs from the "pay and spay" facilities. The different age brackets of the patients that access the programs require different bundles to be established, based on practice philosophy and the clients' awareness of state-of-the-art technology. Some practices have used the national pet health insurance program (DVM/VPI) to offer a Level B coverage beyond the HMA, similar to a catastrophic healthcare insurance alternative. The DVM/VPI company even offers cancer riders, which for some species, if the practice becomes a patient advocate before the expected oncology condition arises, means an alternative to early euthanasia.

The standard cost of an adult HMA approximates $200 but is often priced slightly less for impact. Credit card charges can be keyed in at two- to four-week intervals over a six-week period of time. A puppy or kitten program cost is generally over $200, so five tickets or checks are used for the same purpose. However, submissions need to be made at two-week intervals to ensure the healthcare does not exceed the cash collected.

Applied Bundling

With the puppy or kitten series of vaccinations, as well as the heartworm or FeLV screening series, the quotables are already being proactively priced individually, so if they can be combined into a bundled series based on multiple visits, which can often be handled by outpatient nurses, the services can be further discounted due to prepayment. In lieu of discounting for prepayment, nutritional counseling with vendor samples or fecal laboratory exams could be added to the practice bundle to differentiate the quality practice's bundled series from the local shot clinic offerings. A sample puppy program is presented in Figure 3.5.

In some practices, the senior's program (people, not animals) simply includes the usual AARP prices, but doctor consultations are longer (30 instead of 20 minutes), and the times are shifted to midday schedule slump

KARNARDLY VETERINARY HOSPITAL "BUNDLED BARGAINS"
The "Preferred" Concerned Client Program
a prepaid program

TOTAL WELLNESS PUPPY PROGRAM	VALUE	PROGRAM COST
Pet Selection/Adoption Consultation	$ 21.50	Courtesy
Doctor's Consultation (6-8 weeks)	$ 21.50	Courtesy
- Distemper Complex Vaccination	$ 14.75	$ 10.25
- Parasite Exams (Internal & External)	$ 9.95	$ 9.95
- Internal Parasite Worming	$ 11.50	$ 7.50
- House Training Consultation	Courtesy	Courtesy
Technician Consultation (9-11 weeks)	$ 14.50	Preferred Client
- Nutritional Counseling	Courtesy	Courtesy
- Distemper Complex Vaccination	$ 14.75	$ 10.25
- Kennel Cough Vaccination	$ 19.90	$ 10.25
- Internal Parasite Worming	$ 11.50	$ 7.50
- Family Socialization Behavior Consult	Courtesy	Courtesy (*)
Technician Consultation (12-14 weeks)	$ 14.50	Preferred Client
- Distemper Complex Vaccination	$ 14.75	$ 10.25
- Kennel Cough Vaccination	$ 19.90	$ 10.25
- Puppy Behavior Management	$ 15.00	Courtesy
- Parasite Exams (Internal & External)	$ 9.95	Preferred Client
Doctor's Consultation (16-18 weeks)	$ 21.50	$ 14.50
- Rabies Immunization	$ 8.50	$ 6.95
- Parvo Booster	$ 8.50	$ 6.95
	=====	======
TOTAL "NEW PUPPY" COST	$252.45	$104.60 (**)

(*) This second vaccination will give our preferred clients primary access to our puppy club or kitten carrier class, a once per week evening meeting to assist in the socialization and training needs of these new "members" in the family. See the attached flyer for more details.

*(**) The preferred client is one who takes the best care of this new family member. We want to recognize this special person by ALSO providing a **$25 credit** for our community's pet population control spay and neuter program. This $25 will be deducted from the surgery expense of a spay or neuter for this pet if the surgery appointment is made between the ages of five and seven months (we try to do this surgery before the first "heat" cycle, the least traumatic time for the young animal).*

Fig. 3.5. Sample puppy program incorporating bundling.

periods—seniors like the social time! It is more common to see practices pursue the older pet, with a desire to establish a baseline of information. This effort is often too expensive for a single visit, so it lends itself to multiple visits and has become a method of bundling. For instance, geriatric patient may be treated in the Senior Friends Wellness Program (here, senior refers to the owner, not the pet) or the Arthritis Program. These are practice-specific programs: in a senior citizen area, the Senior Friends Wellness Program is effective, and in a common mixed catchment area, the fall Arthritis Program works well since the cooler damp air of fall makes the clients perceive a locomotion problem that the practice offers to resolve. Once an elderly animal is treated by the practice, the care is stair stepped, such as "Let us take X rays today, including the 'over-40' cardiac pictures, and then I will call you and we will evaluate what needs to be done next." In any preventive care program for a healthy aging animal, a screening lab test for internal organ function (less than $50), a screening Lead 2 ECG for less than $20, or even a screening joint X ray (less than $50) can be used to initiate the diagnostic process. The logical reason for senior pet care is simple. In an illness-related aging pet presentation, the practice needs to first determine the blood chemistry values, identify the standard ECG tracing for the patient, and develop the thoracic/abdominal screening film; these early baselines established during the preventive care can be use for later comparisons. Dental care may or may not be part of the baseline, since this is very practice dependent. Remember, with the aging animal, a doctor can treat pain, but only the client can perceive the suffering. This concept needs to be introduced early in the process so clients know they have a significant role in the evaluation process.

The Senior Friends Wellness Program should be offered in three formats: (1) all baselines will be established today on an inpatient basis, (2) the baseline will be established over the next three weeks, or (3) the elements will be established monthly over this next quarter to reduce the stress on the patient. The option for no is not offered, but the clients are made aware that they may waive the care or defer the decision until the next visit. The wellness of their pets is their decision.

Is This Bundle for You?

Prepayment is one way to guarantee a client's return, but there is also a danger in establishing expectations that cannot rationally be met by the practice. As such, emergency procedures, X rays, ECGs (except for geriatric screening), and similar services are usually not included within a bundled program. In pricing, it is also important not to discount a specific service within a bundled wellness package. A practice does not want to give the impression of being routinely overpriced, so discounting the bundle needs to be specifically justified by the client's prepayment or full compliance. Asking the client to pay before services are rendered is a good reason to discount higher than the local community's IRA savings account interest rates (usually the discount for bundling services is 10–15 percent).

Bundling services can be internally marketed as Special Pet Wellness

Programs of the practice. Some practices call them Preferred Client Programs or Concerned Client Programs, names similar to those used for human healthcare programs. Whatever they're called, all are based on patient advocacy and compassionate care, that is, telling clients what is needed for quality wellness and companion animal protection. Bundling services are also client centered, allowing clients who want the best for their pets to access quality care for a lower cost, if possible. Let the clients decide which is best for them—paying over time at a higher total rate or prepayment for a lower rate (which commits them to returning to your practice for a longer period of time).

The decision to bundle services is practice dependent and must fit the philosophy of the practice as well as the comfort zone of the practitioners.

Bill Balaban—It Pays to Care

Interacting with animals benefits our health and well-being.
—Delta Society

Let me introduce you to a friend, Bill Balaban; he is a pet owner. Being a pet owner, he has the information each practitioner needs to hear. Each practice needs to solicit information from patrons, directly or through client surveys, focus groups, or a Council of Clients. This chapter closes with Bill's very special perspective, since he has been active in the Delta Society (he created the Assistance Animal Awards) and, more recently, he helped start the Center for Animals in Society (University of California, Davis). He has a deep interest in the veterinary profession, as shown by the annual scholarship he funds, which is named for a companion animal of his. He is also an active member of the California Veterinary Medical Association and sits on two of its committees. His previous vocation shapes his presentations: he was a television producer/director and understands the emotions of the American consumer.

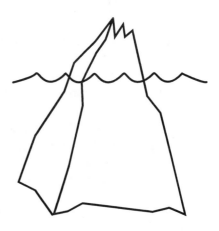

His Questions

At an annual Delta Society meeting in Saint Louis, Bill asked some very interesting questions one evening. We were discussing assistance animals and the unique needs of their owners, but what I heard Bill talking about was the needs of the elderly, as well as a physically challenged, client.

"Why doesn't every practice package multiple prescriptions in different type containers, even if it means just wrapping a rubber band around one of two pill vials?" Clients need a way to remember the difference, especially if they can't see well.

"Why does a practice just talk louder when someone can't hear well, instead of writing the instructions to ensure the client understands?" Effective communication gets the client to return, and return visits are the lifeblood of practices today.

"When an animal needs to be alert, whether it be a seeing eye dog or just a pet that cannot be carried, why does a practice use drugs that make the animal nonresponsive or incapable of effective locomotion and then release the pet to the owner?" The client who must manhandle a pet home from the veterinarian's feels the practice does not care, and he or she will seek one that does for the next visit.

"Why do practices charge for an annual physical but only do a cursory exam? I get an annual physical and want the doctor to tell me if something is changing; why don't veterinarians examine the pet so I can be told what is really needed to keep my pet healthy?" This is especially true for aging animals as well as for puppies and kittens who are getting shots; practices are not offering affordable value and needed services. A new puppy can have behavior management training at the second and third vaccination visit instead of just receiving another physical exam (the client will be appreciative, especially if house-training is the focus). Owners of elderly animals deserve to be offered a laboratory evaluation to start their pets' golden years program. These services will also show that you care about their animals as more than just patients.

It was interesting to listen to Bill, especially when he said it is an insult to be offered a discount just because he has grey hair. He is an A client who sees the world of veterinary medicine full of opportunities not being taken advantage of by most practices. He told me about the veterinary practice he patronizes. It was just sold to a husband and wife team. He observed the following.

"All their prices immediately went up by the computer's incremental percentage program, so vaccinations are now $17.42; don't they know how stupid that seems to a consumer?" Bill understands the need for his veterinarians to make a reasonable profit and increase their prices, he just doesn't understand the logic of across-the-board changes without thought to volume and inventory turnover.

"I now must wait in the examination room only to be rushed through the examination process and treatment. Why don't they explain what they are doing? Why don't they provide a running commentary, of good and bad, so

I can know what they are finding? Or if they do say something, why do they speak in 'medicalese'?" The more good news that is shared during the physical exam, the more likely the client will want to correct those few atypical findings and also make them "good news." This technique has been advocated by consultants for a long time.

"Why don't veterinarians understand their technicians are nurses and use them as nurses, allowing them to give shots and do the wellness screens?" They could transfer the client's confidence to the tech and concurrently enable the practice to be more efficient. It seems to me it would be good business! This client observation made me smile, since the outpatient technician concept seems to be one area where my consulting team has been trying to break a profession paradigm for ages, and we are still changing practices only one at a time.

Bill talks about veterinarians he has known, those who have taken the time to talk to him as a person and the one who wouldn't let him go home after a middle-of-the-night emergency seizure episode until he calmed down (it took a drink of scotch in the veterinarian's apartment, which was above the practice). Bill would wait forever to see these veterinarians: he knew they cared; they knew he cared. They had a bond.

The Bond

Clients have a bond with their pets. My original research on the animal's role in the family (*The Pet Connection,* CENSHARE, University of Minnesota) showed that 75 percent of pets were given family member status and a third of those were given people status. This becomes interesting when you realize that, in almost every practice, when clients are told of a pet need, about 75 percent accept the offered service or product. This bond can be exploited by money hungry veterinarians, and if it is, the client will generally feel violated and change practices.

The client-patient-veterinarian bond isn't a new concept; even the FDA requires it! The international organization that focuses on the interrelationship of people, animals, and the environment is the Delta Society (800-869-6898); it has been trying to share ideas about it with our profession for over a decade, yet most veterinarians don't have the time to listen. The veterinarians are trying too hard to make ends meet and, like usual, are stepping over dollars to pick up

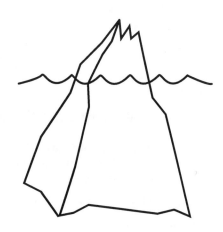

pennies. In fact, Bill Balaban says he stays away from practices where the owners are between 4 and 20 years out of school; he feels this group is too focused on the cash flow and doesn't have time to recognize the bond. New graduates remember why they entered veterinary school and still get the warm feelings and rewards from the bond itself, and by the time veterinarians are over 20 years in practice, they have accepted their position in life and return to their roots, the human-animal bond.

Bill is carrying the word to whoever will listen. The California Veterinary Medical Association asked him to sit on two committees to add the client's perspective. The University of California, Davis, veterinary teaching hospital uses Bill to give the students a client's perspective in an ethics seminar. Bill has offered to go anywhere and talk to any veterinary group, student or VMA, usually at his own expense. He sincerely wants to help reestablish the human-animal bond, to increase sensitivity to the assistance animal owner needs, and to carry his client awareness message. If a client like Bill has this perception of our profession, wouldn't it be smart to find out what your practice's clients are feeling?

The practice must first build the bond, taking the time to find out about the clients and their desires. This is why an extra 10 minutes should be added to all new clients' appointment time; this additional time is for listening, not extra doctor talking. Give the elderly an extra 10 minutes, instead of a 10 percent discount, and promote it as "we don't want to rush you—we want to give you the time to ask all your questions."

When at least 75 percent of clients will accept a presurgical laboratory screen, a heartworm blood test, a dental prophy, or even an allergy-testing procedure, it does not mean these people are waiting to be fleeced. Clients want affordable value; they want to use their discretionary income to the maximum benefit. The practice that understands that each client has different needs, just as each pet has different needs, will become more successful. This same practice records client responses in the progress notes so there will be a continuity of care at the next visit. If a veterinarian can start a "needs" conversation where it left off during the last visit, the chances of the client's pet receiving improved care increases. The more return visits, the better the care, the greater the cash flow. Yes my friends, it does pay to care!

Puppy Club and Kitten Carrier Classes

The puppy club and kitten carrier classes are examples of ways practices can bond with clients and their pets. The puppy club has many formats, but the most exciting is the one conducted by the veterinary practice's paraprofessional team. It is an opportunity for the staff to help clients become better stewards of their companion animals. They meet with clients and pets in the evening, for 60 minutes maximum, since puppies have a 15-minute maximum tolerance. The kitten carrier class is an extension of this concept, since we want the owners of all critters to bond to the practice through this "value-added" service. Kitten and puppy classes should meet on different nights.

The classes are formatted around the expertise of your staff. Socialization means simply getting the animals used to coming to the practice when they aren't receiving an injection. Besides adjusting to other animals, getting used to being handled by other people, and becoming accustomed to traveling by car, the benefits of these classes are

1. Helping the owners deal with feet (nails), ears (plucking and cleaning), tails (anals), teeth (brushing), and other anatomically awkward appendages.

2. Discussions about parasites (prevention as well as control), nutrition (diets and treats), and behavior management (e.g., Gentle Leader— Promise head collars).

3. Floor work by group for puppies. Try to keep the class members (puppies) within five weeks of age of each other. The simplest of concepts are used only for 10–15 minutes at a time; then the puppies are allowed to "rest" while other subjects are discussed with the owners.

Some practices provide "two admission tickets—each a $15 value" with each puppy or kitten vaccination visit, thereby encouraging the weekly meaningful contact and adding additional value to the vaccination visit. This makes the value of the puppy club or kitten carrier class a specific dollar amount that leads the practice and client into a fee-for-service, staff-operated, behavior management appointment system in the future.

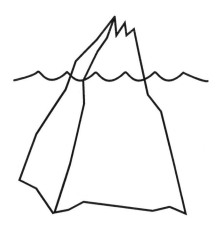

These classes bond the client to the practice, meet the needs of the owner (e.g., 90 percent of new owners desire assistance with behavior management of their pets), and expand the professional image of the practice team. They provide an opportunity to be a leader in your community.

Application Exercise

As stated in the Introduction, mind mapping is an excellent technique not only for generating ideas but also for developing intuitive capabilities. Use the iceberg ideas you have added on the odd-numbered pages and the concepts you have drawn from this chapter to expand the following mind map.

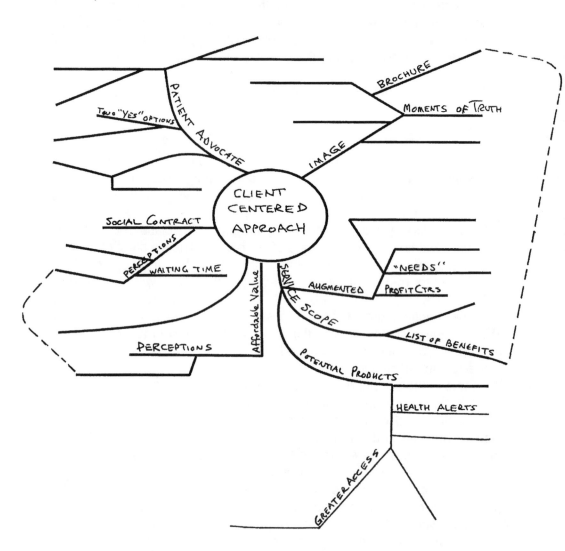

CHAPTER FOUR

Leadership before Delegation

Lead, follow, or get out of the way!

I was leaning back, looking at the Rocky Mountain foothills behind my office, contemplating how to start this "leadership before delegation" application of innovation and creativity, and the phone rang. The person on the other end was a frantic practitioner searching for the ultimate in job descriptions and clinical protocols. His faithful binder of dog-eared standard operating procedures (SOPs) was 10 years old, and the consultant who sold it to him had left the business. He was out-of-date and needed to buy a current set. Catanzaro & Associates stocks many samples and has developed more sets than I wish to remember, but never once have we "sold the answer." I tried to explain the methods we use, where samples are provided to staff and the staff are mentored on how to update their procedures. In fact, when we have an active in-service training program, the staff generally demand an ongoing update. The practitioner did not understand—he just wanted to have a piece of paper to solve the problems of the day. So we built an "ASK SOP" diagram while on the phone and mailed it to him. It initially looked something like Figure 4.1.

But this was not the reasonable adaptation of what I was trying to explain. This is what most practices embrace when they first try an interactive leadership method and expose their staff and practices to the chaos of change. As I explored leadership in Volume 1 of this series, and applied those skills to programs and procedures in Volume 2, I tried to keep the knowledge-skills-attitude relationship (the iceberg) in perspective. After my conversation with the frantic practitioner, I added direction to the elements in Figure 4.1 to expand the relationship of practice leadership to success (see arrow change, Figs. 4.1 and 4.2), and I adjusted the principles of the "ASK the SOP" scenario:

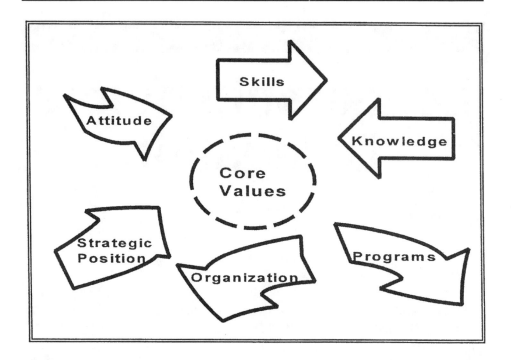

Fig. 4.1. ASK SOP diagram, version 1.

ATTITUDE   We hire for attitude. Team fit and belief
                                     are a must!

SKILLS   Skills are reflected in life experiences
                                     and ability to perform during the orienta-
                                     tion phase.

KNOWLEDGE   Knowledge is understanding why and
                                     asking to learn more.

STRATEGIC ORIENTATION   Strategic orientation includes market
                                     niche, new services, client outreach,
                                     and a smile.

ORGANIZATION STRUCTURE   Organization structure includes job re-
                                     design and outcome accountabilities,
                                     among other things.

PROGRAMS AND ACTIVITIES   The cash is only the score card. Service
                                     is key.

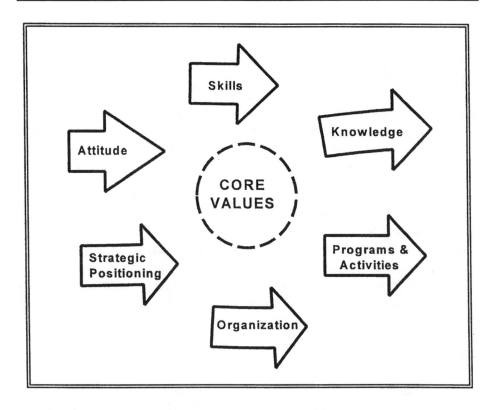

Fig. 4.2. ASK SOP diagram, revised.

The Path of Reason

The last words of a dying practice:
"We never did it that way!"

My experience with the SOP-dependent practitioner was not unlike that of a leadership course I was staffing, the summer of 1994, in the New Mexico Rockies. We had picked up the participants Saturday morning and led them to the base camp at 7,300 feet elevation. We had 24 hours to "shake them down" and get them ready for the trail. There was a dentist from North Carolina

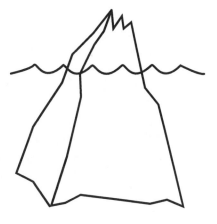

who was tired, had failed in one practice, and was pushing too hard in the current practice he was building. There was also an environmental scientist from Texas, a hulking but nice, quiet guy. The chief operator of Housing for the Aged, from an eastern state, had led youth for 10 years and was burned out. He wanted his excitement to be rekindled. The pediatric surgeon from Dallas had been a Navy Seal in Viet Nam and knew he could survive without the others. He knew he could even survive without this course! The comptroller from an international shipping firm continuously played with his folding knife. The group nicknamed him "the blade." The youngest was in video production. He had owned his own firm since he was 16, seven years ago. He needed to break away from the demands of his family and become his own person. The head engineer of a back east State Highway Planning Commission knew how to use a map and compass and would keep everyone else from getting lost. The architect from Oklahoma was truly a nice guy—so nice that it was hard for him to make hard decisions. The group members all wanted the answers for their future; they thought a week in the backcountry would help clear the cobwebs and that learning new leadership skills would facilitate their success.

Eight in a Group

As the staff facilitator of this group, one of eight groups in the course, my job was to help the members learn leadership skills, to awaken the values and ethics inside each of them, and to give their beliefs some form and structure that could be used to lead others. They were eight individuals who had never met, all from different walks of life, all from different parts of the country, and all with different personal agendas. In many ways, this group was like an average veterinary practice, except we changed the leader each day. The job of group leadership was rotated among the eight, with each being accountable for success for 24 hours.

Time management is a tool used to facilitate group development. The dentist knew he was a bad time manager and expected to fail. The group members cooked their own meals, usually a dehydrated meal that only required heat and water, but the meals had to be ready on time. During the first 24 hours, no meal was on time, the group was never together at the designated time and place to eat, and members felt rushed at every turn. Late on day two, when it was time for a canteen refill from the stream, the eight were ready to go down to the stream. I whispered in the leader's (the dentist's) ear, "How many does it take to carry the canteens down to fill them? If it is less than eight, will others have more time to do other things?" He immediately saw the folly of his do-it-yourself leadership style and suggested only two take all the canteens so the others could stay behind, relax, and work on their trail journals. The group rejoiced at the great new idea of sharing the work and trusting others to do the required job for the good of all. The members applied the same principle to preparing meals, setting up camp, and doing other group duties. They became more efficient and had more time for personal projects. Not unlike a busy veterinary practice.

On the trail, they needed to hike as a group of eight, not as a group of three and another of five, or two and six, or even four and four. Trail safety required a group of eight. They did not do this for the first two days and received negative feedback on the safety hazards they created. If one slipped and fell off the trail down the 100-foot drop to the stream below, it would take at least two to stay and mark the trail point (since a person should never be alone in the mountains), three more to follow down and be with the fallen comrade, and two others to go for help. Response time might be critical for stopping the bleeding, restoring the airway, or just pulling a pack-laden hiker from the rushing mountain water. It would be the responsibility of each to watch out for the others, for safety as well as for success, so they needed to be together. Not unlike a veterinary practice staff.

Near the end of day two on the trail, this developing team came upon another group stopped at a rushing stream. The spring runoff had washed out the log bridges, and there was no dry way across the icy stream. Immediately my group decided to build a bridge for the others, and while it was building the bridge, three other groups amassed on the bank, waiting for a dry way to cross. The bridge was built, and the four groups crossed, thanking the bridge builders. This "bridge building for self and others" recurred three more times that afternoon, before the group reached the night camp site. The members were delayed in reaching their destination, but they felt good about what they had done. The following morning at assembly, three of the groups publicly recognized the bridge builders. The group had become a team by helping others, and this team would not be separated ever again. We have seen this occur in veterinary practices, especially in those very difficult cases requiring a team effort. It feels good!

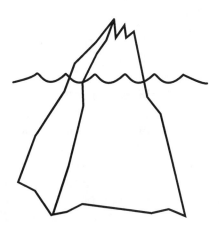

A Team of Eight

The team planned what needed to be done, shared the accountability for the outcomes (not the process), and had more time to do new things. When the members wrote a plan in their trail journals, they automatically wrote a second or third plan, in case unforeseen problems derailed the first idea. Failure gave way to innovation. "We never did it that way" gave way to "Let's try a new way." The team's expectation became to exceed the traditional expectations. The team's tenacity and creativity were being recognized by others, and the team pride grew.

On day four, the first trail task was to find the staff at a mountain ridge that had been pinpointed on their maps the night before. The eight groups were not to use any roads but otherwise could get there however they wanted. The same location was given to all of the groups, with an arrival time of 9:30 a.m. being part of the parameters. The staff left early so no one could follow them. The eight groups had sight of each other, and one started to go up a jeep trail. The bridge builders followed for a few hundred yards but then stopped. They realized the map wasn't completely correct, new roads had been built, so they reassessed their plan. Four groups continued up the jeep road while this group looked for alternatives. The bridge builders decided to backtrack to the last trail crossing and reassess their route from there. By going back, they found the appropriate trail, took it, and arrived at the ridge with time to spare. The four groups on the jeep trail arrived 90 minutes late. By stopping to reassess, by going back to a previous turning point, by not following the crowd, the bridge builders had gained efficiency and success. They were happy hikers.

The Right Path

The right path for any team is the route the team needs to take to achieve its dream. The vision of the leader must paint the trail markers. The path to success is often obscured by markers left by others. Detours abound. But the leadership task is clear:

1. Decide where it is important to focus your efforts; have clarity of purpose.

2. Decide what resources will be needed to get to that goal and commit them.

3. Make the commitment to action and act decisively.

4. In case of failure, alter the efforts to reach success; don't settle for less.

Many managers are stopped by reduced resources, environmental challenges, more pressing problems, or a host of other excuses. There is only one reason for a leader to stop ... success! A manager has projects and programs; a leader has a team. True leaders get things done through other people, by a group effort. The skilled manager has taught all group members exactly how to do their jobs, regularly appraises their compliance, and often scores them on a scale of 1 to 10, with 10 being the best. The leader teaches the skill, then persuades the team member to accept accountability, then coaches to ensure appropriate behavior is reinforced. Only then does the leader delegate the outcome, an outcome that the team member can achieve with innovation and creativity, since the member knows the parameters of excellence expected.

The path of reason has room for error for every team member; it allows people to reverse directions and admit mistakes. Celebration replaces chastisement. There is no such thing as a level 10 team member to a true leader. There is no such thing as perfection. Every person needs to be learning each day, even the leader. The path of reason has inverted speed bumps—some may call them the potholes of life—but they are there to allow creativity while ensuring the pace remains reasonable. After successful delegation, the leader becomes a consultant to the team and, when possible, joins with the group to participate in the toils. A great leader understands that new tasks require new training, more persuading, and additional coaching before new delegation occurs. The leader also understands that a new group member requires that the group be reformed into a new and different team. On the path of reason, time spent on training and group development is never seen as wasted time; it is necessary for success.

The path of reason is not a busy trail, so the landmarks are sometimes hard to see. There are signs of decay at the edges of the path, where some have lost their dreams and direction to a distraction off the trail. The path of reason isn't a jeep trail through the mountains. It is an individual vision quest of a leader who shows the way to others. As one mountain plateau is reached by the team, a new one is identified by the leader. The team is kept together, and the tasks and skills are divided equitably based on individual abilities to learn and develop. The rewards of the path of reason are feelings of greatness and compassion and team pride.

As the bridge builder's ex–Navy Seal said at the end of the week, with tears in his eyes, "I have never felt so close to a group of guys since Viet Nam," and my reply was, "I know." May your path of reason make you feel this good about your team.

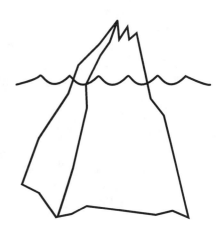

Mistakes of the Mind

A decision is an action an executive must take when he has information so
incomplete that the answer does not suggest itself.
—Arthur Radford

As I visit hundreds of veterinary practices, it is interesting to observe the mind-set of specific key leaders. Trite phrases abound: "It won't work," "That's not our style," "It's too late," "We can't ...," " "If only ...," and "Yes, but ..." When we only look backward in time, we will repeat history. When we dwell on what could have been, we get no further. There is more than one mind-set that causes this backward thinking.

Flawed Leadership

Veterinarians who make too many management decisions are those who do not use their staff services very well. Anyone can make decisions. Just ask the kennel man if you should buy a new computer or not, and you'll get an answer. But this is not a decision; it is a guess. Most good decisions are self-evident based on the research and background knowledge of the hospital staff. Fear of failure often stops a project before it starts; the quick-draw no by the boss kills the evil change before it has a chance to see the light of day and be tested. The best practice leaders promote change by *requiring* a 90-day test, established and coordinated by the staff members who proposed the idea, before evaluation by the leadership team.

Another common alternative to the fast-draw no is the management excuse based on "superior experience." This is common with doctors, but it is more common with tenured staff who are comfortable in the old ways and unwilling to make the personal changes needed to support the practice. We can call these types of attitudes many things, but in this text, we shall just term them the dirty dozen stagnation philosophies.

The Dirty Dozen Stagnation Philosophies

1. Disqualifying: *"That couldn't be implemented here."*
2. Editing: *"That is a great idea but won't work in this area."*
3. All-or-nothing thinking: *"If we can't do it 100 percent, we won't try it."*
4. Acceptance of critics: *"They have said it isn't smart."*
5. Perfectionism: *"I need more information on how to ensure success."*
6. Fortune-telling: *"I'll never get my clients to accept that."*

7. Overgeneralization: *"If we did that we would not have time to breathe."*
8. Emotional reasoning: *"I know we'd never be happy doing it that way."*
9. Labeling: *"That is unethical advertising."*
10. Personalization: *"If I did that my colleagues would ..."*
11. Minimizing: *"We could try it but it wouldn't make a great difference."*
12. Complacency: *"I am happy with what I've done to get here, so we don't need to change."*

Eliminate Excuses

Many things get in the way of doing a function as it ought to be done: work overload, understaffing, too many bosses, being short on resources, too many rules, not enough experience, improper training, ineffective leadership, and so on. Staff members also may come to the practice handicapped with personal problems or lack of a proper attitude. It is impossible to eliminate all the factors that may make it difficult for a staff member to do a superior job. But it is possible to help that person become more productive in spite of those factors.

Practices that blame external circumstances for practice problems, such as staff conflicts or slowed growth, do not look for solutions. They prequalify failure. As they say in the dairy industry, "Don't cry over spilt milk; just find another cow to milk."

Problems prevent good performance only when they become excuses for not trying to improve. Use the phrase "given that ..." when you address the next set of excuses you hear. Using it, you will acknowledge real handicaps yet insist the staff member find a way to be more productive despite those challenges; this statement is a powerful way to remove the excuse so that a productive discussion about how to improve performance can occur.

A common excuse is "the clients can't afford that level of care; you are offering Cadillac care to a Yugo population." In reply, think about saying, "I know it would be easier if every client loved a pet like a family member and had the money to keep it in perfect health, but given that clients don't, what can be done to bring the standard of preventive and forensic medicine offerings up to a level that helps the pet and still considers the economic plight of the clients?"

"Given that" statements eliminate long and unproductive discussions about how bad things are or about whether or not a staff member is justified in being frustrated. They also put the responsibility back on the staff member not to allow handicaps to serve as excuses for not trying to improve performance.

Bottom Line

In the case of excuses, one item remains constant: the target must be well-defined by the leadership of the practice. No member of the staff can be expected to pursue the practice goals if they are kept a secret, remain ill-defined, or are not put into measurable terms. If the ownership decides to target a certain level of healthcare as the standard, then that is the measurement that must be used. Excuses contrary to that goal need to be eliminated.

We have discussed methods to eliminate the mental mistakes that become detrimental habits, but some staff members will not respond to coaching, discussion, or even "given that" acknowledgments. An astute manager must realize that they are probably at the wrong practice, and maybe even in the wrong profession. A good leader will help those staff members who want assistance in learning how to reach the practice target and will eliminate those who won't accept it.

Mistakes of the mind include having all the answers or believing someone else has them, such as a practice consultant. There is no guarantee that any one consultant's ideas will work better than yours; however, a good consultant can tailor ideas to your practice by using the lessons learned from successful practice management assistance. Challenge all assumptions and use the power within your team to assess the reality of a new idea. If you have the intestinal fortitude to take the chance with your own team, to trust their opinions, the innovation engine will fire up within your practice. Many ideas will fail of their own accord, and others will be modified in the implementation process; for the ones that survive, be prepared for the resultant creativity, team synergy, and success.

A Trio of Leadership Principles

In the first volume of *Building the Successful Veterinary Practice: Leadership Tools,* I shared the concept that there are three group-forming skills. After these three group-forming leadership skills are addressed and implemented, then and only then can we proceed with group activities:

- Knowing and using the resources of the group
- Effective communication
- Understanding the characteristics and needs of the group

Knowing and using the resources of the group means that every brain in the group is a valuable asset to nurture and cherish. Each person brings new perspectives and impressions that will help the group proceed and prosper. The community calendar, professional associations, clubs, time, money, written references, animals, vendors, audio-visual aids, friends, and clients are other resources that must be developed as potential practice assets. The Council of Clients (discussed in Chapter Three) is an example of one valuable resource: clients know what they want and also know what they perceive they can get from the practice, and these are not always the same. There is no one to blame for this perspective except ourselves if we don't use the available resources to the very best of our ability as practice leaders.

Effective communication is most simply defined as the giving and getting of meaningful information. But it is not that simple in a veterinary practice. Our patients have an abundance of information to share, but we get it only if we use the appropriate diagnostics. Clients communicate with us by words, voice tones, body language, or just not coming back through the door. If we "listen" to these nonverbal messages, we can usually make the proper decisions. This also applies to the nonverbal exchanges of staff, family, and friends of every member of the practice team. Data must be processed to become meaningful. A urine pH of 5.5 in a dog is a message that must be interpreted; it is not an answer.

A hospital's expensive veterinary software program may tell us in very finite detail about income and how clients spend money, but unless it is tied to an expense-monitoring program for similar centers of activity, we do not know if we are earning a profit. A leader must be aware of all messages being sent, verbal and nonverbal, and integrate them with the environment to ensure effective communication occurs.

Understanding the characteristics and needs of the group is an exciting concept once everyone understands the difference between characteristics and needs. While a characteristic may change with age or the environmental pressures, it should be considered a constant (e.g., poor vision, positive attitudes, hair color, body size, etc.) that causes a series of *needs*:

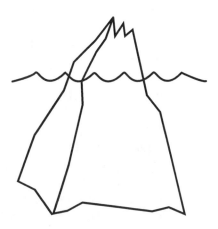

- A person with poor vision needs glasses or lenses, glasses need cleaning, cleaning devices need changing, etc.
- A person with a positive attitude needs feedback, a person providing feedback

needs a safe environment, a safe environment needs individual nurturing, individual nurturing needs collaboration, etc.
- A person who is obese needs to diet, a diet needs to based on the basic food groups, eating a balanced diet from the basic food groups means the dieter needs to be disciplined, etc.

Leaders who consider others' characteristics take off their shoes before walking a single step in those of another; they are aware of others' values and experiences. Leaders who consider others' needs help them find the shoes in which they can walk (job redesign), or the best routes (training), or even the freedom to find their own routes (performance planning).

The Reality

Practices that meet the needs of the client keep the client. Practices that do not will lose the client to someone else who promises to meet the needs. The client may return if the new source does not meet his or her expectations (quality is relative). The superstore or discount clinic only takes those clients who feel they are paying more than what they should for the services provided. Some clients judge practices based only on price, and we caused that with our long line of quotable services. We aggravated it by publishing prices instead of services in the local media. The uninformed consumer of any service or product will judge only by price. The informed consumer considers value when making a decision.

Again, practices must be aware of the *resources* of the group. The client has only discretionary income to spend on a pet (about 11 percent of the take-home dollar). The client has limited time for veterinary visits, often only evenings or weekends in heavy commuting communities. The client has limited knowledge and will judge by price unless educated. It requires *effective communication* to talk to the client in terms he or she can understand. Explaining a handout or brochure before giving it to a client adds value, especially when the client is told, "Here is a handout that explains what we just discussed, in case anybody at home wants to learn more." The doctor states a need for the animal and then listens to the response from the client (and in smart, continuity of care, client-centered practices, the doctor also records the reply in the medical record). This is called getting and giving information. But the animal's *characteristics* (age, sex, vaccination status, condition, etc.) are what causes the *need* for diagnostics, medicines, or other treatment. The client's characteristics (knowledge, discretionary income, bias, etc.) drive the decision to meet the needs. Clients make their decisions based on emotion, and if the provider is not aware of the emotional characteristics of the clients, he or she will not meet the clients' emotional needs. When a veterinarian *understands the character-*

istics and needs of clients and staff, the practice can fulfill them. It is no one's fault if we are not aware, since the skill is not being taught in veterinary school, technician training, or even receptionist training. However, the leader is accountable.

Practice leaders must center on what they can control. They cannot control humane society boards. They cannot control public corporations. They cannot control the characteristics of the individual, but they can meet the needs resulting from those characteristics. Leaders can create the environment for motivation and creativity; only the individual can become motivated. The leader can kill the collaboration required for a team's success or nurture the feedback process by accepting everyone's ideas as acceptable alternatives to meet practice expectations.

> *The leader gives credit and takes blame,*
> *while the manager gives blame and takes credit.*

> *Leaders do the right things, while managers do things right.*

> *If you blame others, you have abdicated control of the resolution.*

The Compliment

Repeatedly, studies report that many Americans admit discomfort, defensiveness, and/or cynicism about compliments and their givers. Yet they still seem to crave praise.

> *A compliment is like a kiss through a veil.*
> —*Victor Hugo*

Coupled with a smile, a sincere compliment is a verbal pat on the back that lets us know that we are appreciated and make us feel good about ourselves and life in general.

A Descriptive Taxonomy

Dr. Mark Knapp, University of Texas, has studied the effects of compliments on more than 500 people; he analyzed over 768

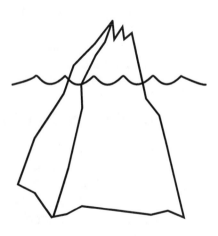

compliments. As reported in the *Journal of Communication,* people found it difficult to take compliments only one-third of the time. The rest of the time, they knew how to deal with them. The explanation lies in the definition (taxonomy) of a compliment and the perceived accuracy of the commendation.

By definition, a compliment is positive. As Knapp defined it, "A compliment is a statement which makes a person believe that they have received a positive evaluation. It can be about performance, appearance, or thoughts, but it must be a positive evaluation for it to be a compliment." The sincerity and veracity of compliments are occasionally challenged. The fancy term used by psychologists to describe these exceptions is the degree of fit. If the compliment does not coincide with what the receiver perceives as truth or if there is little similarity between the compliment and the behavior, then both the compliment and the person who gave it are discredited.

Additionally, if effusive compliments are repeatedly given over a period of time for the most ordinary behaviors, other problems can develop. Recipients no longer discredit the compliments or the people who give them; instead they suspect their own abilities. They believe very few compliments and begin to believe that all of their achievements are overestimated—even the ones that genuinely deserve praise. This dramatically affects their self-esteem.

Knapp found that in any group, whether it be the under-30 group or older groups, about 77 percent of compliments are directed within the age group. In status groups, about 71 percent of the compliments were directed toward colleagues who are equal to them on the corporate ladder; 22 percent to those above them; and 7 percent to those below their defined status level. Sixty percent of all compliments are directed toward members of the same gender. Men tend to compliment both genders equally, but women compliment other women more often than they do men. The key area of unbalance in compliments is in the area of appearance; 78 percent of the compliments received by women are related to appearance, while only 22 percent of the time men receive compliments on attire or image. Compliments on performance, personality, and possessions are balanced between male and female receivers.

The Power of Humble Compliments

Jerald D. Hawkins, EdD, Lander College, believes that compliments are desired by everyone who tries to perform well and should be given when earned. Yet many managers and coaches use criticism for feedback almost exclusively. He believes these types of controlling supervisors see praise as a form of complacency that will make them lose their edge as motivators.

However, in addition to motivational aspects, very positive side effects emerge from giving and accepting a compliment based on performance. After the initial blush and thank-you, individuals disclose more about themselves and work more closely with the compliment giver. This starts a compliment cycle, which includes positive voice inflections, less disagreement, and more cooperation. Hawkins has offered the following guidelines to guarantee that compliments will be accepted:

1) Keep It Simple—Make sure that the compliment conveys only one message. Never use the word "but"; a negative compliment is called criticism.

2) Be Honest—Give accurate appraisals and they will be believable. If it is too far removed from the person's belief, the compliment will be discredited as will your opinion.

3) Do It Immediately—Timing is important to make excitement a beneficial part of the process.

4) Do It Yourself—Don't wait for someone else to do it and don't make the person beg or fish for your opinion. Take the initiative and start the compliment cycle for anyone who deserves it; never worry if the person is your equal in the pecking order.

5) Move from Big to Little—Suggesting you generally admire a person is difficult to refute. Deal with the totality of the person at first, and as you get to know the person, move from general to specific.

6) Mean What You Say—Be prepared to explain the reasons for the compliment if they challenge you. While a few people do this to hear more compliments, you show that the opinions were real, current, and accurate.

No matter what happens in a compliment exchange, one truth remains: the receiver will never walk away unaffected. In most cases, even a false compliment is better than no compliment at all. This is especially true while building a practice team when you need to "catch" people doing things right on a daily basis. The text by Milo Frank, *How to Get Your Point Across in 30 Seconds,* recommended in Volume 1 of *Building the Successful Veterinary Practice* as a critical book for your practice library, deserves review as you accept the chal-

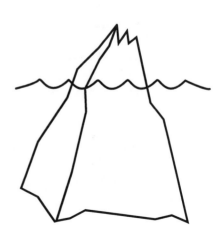

lenge to sincerely acknowledge each team member's effort each week. This is how you build stars on your practice team.

A Star Is Found

Developing a staff to become leaders is often seen as a passive practice task—many feel leaders are born, not made. However, fostering leadership skills is not as difficult as many hospital directors believe. As in basketball, not everyone will be an NBA player, but everyone can learn to play better.

Emerging Behaviors

Some staff members will inevitably emerge as leaders. The veterinary practice challenge is to spot them early and to have them buy into the practice goals and objectives. While there is no magic prescription, good leaders share six behavior patterns that can be used by the astute practice manager:

1. They challenge the process, search for opportunities to institute change, and are restless to make things better. ACTION: Play to their curiosity, challenge their up-to-date knowledge, allow them to query the business-as-usual environment. Many of these prospective leaders are less than ideal as veterinary practice team members since they are not always content in a follower's role.

2. They are good learners who aren't afraid to err, then adapt accordingly. ACTION: Allow them to try new things and make mistakes without embarrassing them. Without this latitude, the staff member won't take the risks that leadership demands.

3. They inspire a shared vision and get other people excited about their ideas. ACTION: Help these people to learn to communicate their ideas in a stimulating manner. Allow them to use their inspirational stories or tales about other successes in veterinary medicine. Incorporate practice goals and objectives into their dreams and place their focus on practice upgrades.

4. They enable other staff members to act by making them feel powerful; they win followers rather than subordinates. They don't always insist on having their way, even when they are right. ACTION:

Acknowledge good ideas from all staff members, encourage brainstorming with a third person rather than engaging in any one-on-one debate, and support group efforts that seem spontaneous yet still good for the practice.

5. They serve as models, realizing that they are always on stage and that leadership is a dramatic art. ACTION: Support their credibility, keep the focus on project completion, show that you trust them to do as planned for the good of the practice, clients, patients, and/or staff.

6. They display the heart and courage to persist. They are unabashed cheerleaders for their projects, they thank people for their contributions, and they build camaraderie. They show the ability to balance the demands of work with their social and personal lives. ACTION: Keep a sense of humor, use a smile to break the tension, support the celebration of team accomplishments.

Shaping Strategies

There are many strategies to develop the staff of a practice into better leaders. While the methods must fit the philosophy of the practice and the scope of services, there are a few that seem to remain constant:

- Delegate to them. Provide varying tasks and job experiences so that they exercise a variety of skills.
- Challenge them. Extend your staff to their limit, but not beyond. People learn to lead through hardship, through the mud, mire, and gunfire of a hectic practice. Unless they are given a chance to tackle tough assignments, you can't make an assessment of how much they can do.
- Allow mistakes. The two best teachers are trial and error. You must allow your staff to make mistakes, even to fail, but you must also be there to pick them up and discuss how to turn the experience into a learning success.

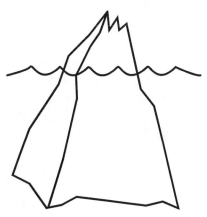

Top Downs

If the controls are too tight, the staff are unlikely to take chances. If you are out to develop leaders who can help your practice grow, you have to be ready to handle a lot more chaos. When people are pushed to the limits of their comfort zones, the system's structure may temporarily suffer. But a good practice will benefit in the long run as capable leaders emerge on your staff.

The character of the staff relationship to clients directly reflects the hospital director's attitude toward the staff. If the staff are simply "my girls" or "the gals up front," the director is projecting an image that is preventing the staff from developing. The entire top-down relationship must be based on mutual respect. The director must foster professional growth and encourage staff to take on practice problems and change them to practice successes. Managers want to control the present based on the past, but leaders have the vision for tomorrow. If you aren't willing to do more than what it took to get you where you are today, the practice will stagnate.

Motivation Excitement

Leaders create environments that allow motivation,
while managers only cause perspiration.
—Dr. T. E. Cat

As a volunteer leader in community programs, you need to know how to motivate those who offer to work for free. Much has been written on methods to recognize the contributions of volunteers, but seldom does someone tell you how to motivate them. In veterinary practices where the staff members are dedicated and work for low wages, the advice that does exist for motivating volunteers applies to staff as well.

Motivation Analysis

During my Baylor study toward a master's in healthcare administration, I discovered D. C. McClelland and J. W. Atkinson had developed a series of 11 questions a few years earlier that allowed an evaluator to class volunteers into three different motivational groups to find the "hot buttons" for volunteers. Since we constantly look for ways to push our staff members' hot buttons or at least to get their attention, these questions (Fig. 4.3) are applicable to a veterinary practice—especially since the wages most practices pay almost equate their staff to volunteer status!

McClelland and Atkinson's system is simply to seek volunteers' preferences in specific situations and then to use those replies to determine their real tendencies (what makes them feel good). While we can design our healthcare delivery system to use the specific strengths of our staff, and

Each of the following groups has three choices. Choose the one statement (place an "X" before the letter) that makes you feel MOST comfortable; there are NO wrong answers.

1. __a. When doing a job, I seek feedback.
   __b. I prefer to work alone and am eager to be my own boss.
   __c. I seem to be uncomfortable when forced to work alone.

2. __a. I go out of my way to make friends with new people.
   __b. I enjoy a good argument.
   __c. After starting a task, I am not comfortable until it is completed.

3. __a. Status symbols are important to me.
   __b. I am always getting involved in group projects.
   __c. I work better when there is a deadline.

4. __a. I work best when there is some challenge involved.
   __b. I would rather give orders than take them.
   __c. I am sensitive to others—especially when they are mad.

5. __a. I am eager to be my own boss.
   __b. I accept responsibility eagerly.
   __c. I try to get personally involved with my superiors.

6. __a. I am uncomfortable when given a task to complete by myself.
   __b. I prefer to do it myself, even when others feel a joint effort is required.
   __c. When given responsibility, I set measurable standards of high performance.

7. __a. I am very concerned about my reputation or position.
   __b. I have a desire to out-perform others.
   __c. I am concerned with keeping harmony and being accepted.

8. __a. I enjoy and seek warm, friendly relationships.
   __b. I attempt complete involvement in a project.
   __c. Since I have knowledge, I want my ideas to be accepted.

9. __a. I desire unique accomplishments.
   __b. It concerns me when the tasking isolates me from others.
   __c. I have a need and desire to train others.

10. __a. I think about consoling and helping others.
    __b. I speak very well and communicate effectively.
    __c. I am restless and innovative.

11. __a. I set goals and think about ways to attain them.
    __b. I think about ways to change people.
    __c. I think a lot about my feelings and the feelings of others.

Fig. 4.3. Questions designed to identify what motivates individuals. Developed by D.C. McClelland and J.W. Atkinson.

we can learn how to package our staff taskings to meet their comfort zone, the basic rule to remember for motivation is

Motivation comes from internal sources,

perspiration is from external sources.

There are no right or wrong answers to the questions in Figure 4.3, just personal preferences. Figure 4.4 is the key to categorizing the responses, and Figure 4.5 can be used to plot the results to reveal what motivates an individual. For a practice leader, this test is one gateway into a staff member's inner self.

Circle the word that corresponds to the letter you marked in the exercise; tally the count for each word in the TOTAL COUNT below.

1. a. Achievement b. Power c. Affiliation	7. a. Power b. Achievement c. Affiliation	
2. a. Affiliation b. Power c. Achievement	8. a. Affiliation b. Achievement c. Power	
3. a. Power b. Affiliation c. Achievement	9. a. Achievement b. Affiliation c. Power	
4. a. Achievement b. Power c. Affiliation	10. a. Affiliation b. Power c. Achievement	
5. a. Power b. Achievement c. Affiliation	11. a. Achievement b. Power c. Affiliation	
6. a. Affiliation b. Power c. Achievement		

TOTAL COUNT:

Achievement _____

Power _____

Affiliation _____

Fig. 4.4. Key to categorizing questions in Figure 4.3. Developed by D.C. McClelland and J.W. Atkinson.

Plot the three scores on the lines provided, with "0" being the point of convergence for the three lines, and each dot being one unit as it moves toward the "classification word."

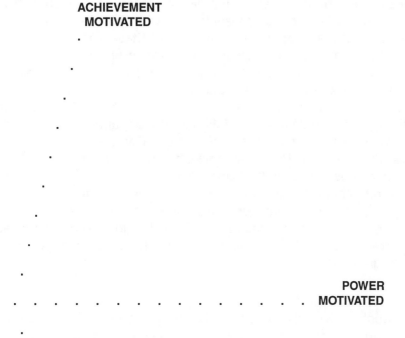

ACHIEVEMENT MOTIVATED

POWER MOTIVATED

The triangle formed by connecting the three dots will reveal an individual's "tendency" toward what motivates him or her. Take this classification back to the "type" descriptions and "light their fire"!

AFFILIATION MOTIVATED

Fig. 4.5. Graph for plotting results of Figure 4.4. Developed by D.C. McClelland and J.W. Atkinson.

Motivation Factors

The three basic categories of hot buttons in McClelland and Atkinson's system are achievement, power, and affiliation. Recent studies on motivation in human healthcare, as presented at the American College of Healthcare Executives, suggest that in the United States recognition is the number one motivator of paraprofessional teams, while belonging is the number one motivator in Europe. That only leaves power unaccounted for, which may be due to the simple fact that only 17 percent of the American workforce has a dominant personality type, while 50 percent has a steady personality type, 17 percent has an influencing type, and 17 percent has a compliance-oriented personality. These personality types can be identified with a DISC Personal Behavior Profile, but that is another process for the practice to consider at another time.

We must remember that most people react to all three motivators, depending on the situation or pressures they are experiencing. A good manager will know which motivators to use in which situations by evaluating an employee's responses to the questions in Figure 4.3. Some common traits within each group are

Achievement motivated

These people have a desire for excellence and want to be recognized for doing a good job. The outcome measurement for projects must be clear and within the initial delegation negotiation for best results. The tasks need to be regarded as important accomplishments, or they must be assigned from the boss. Achievement-motivated individuals want to advance in their careers based on their own merit and want feedback to validate their progress.

    Examples: Inventory management team member
                 Nutritional counselor
                 Animal behavior specialist
                 Client relations manager

Power motivated

These people want to lead and need to give advice or at least be asked an opinion frequently. Clear lines of independent responsibility and authority, as well as budget constraint, work wonders with these folk. The taskings need to be related to the prestige of a title or job status, and they want everyone to recognize them in that role. Power-motivated individuals enjoy influencing people and activities, especially when their ideas can predominate.

Examples: Practice manager
            Paraprofessional manager
            Team leader
            Head receptionist

Affiliation motivated

These people like to be popular and care about what other people think of them. They must be recognized for their efforts in front of their peers for best results. The taskings need to be team efforts where they can be interactive with others, can help others, and be friendly in the process. They dislike being alone in work or play.

Examples: Pet placement specialist
            Technician team member
            Receptionist team member
            Technician assistant

Some practice staff cannot be categorized into the above parameters simply because their leadership styles and/or group development stages do not correspond (see Vol. 1 of this series). There are many other categories of motivation, but since the above three fit most mature practices, we shall proceed from this basis.

Practice Application Techniques

Now that you are armed with this knowledge, it is time to apply it. Some ways to push staff members' hot buttons include

- Hang a changeable letter board in reception that displays each of the staff member's names and titles (even better, framed 8x10-inch pictures of staff with their pets that include the staff members' names and titles as well as the pets' names).
- Assign name tags (they could list first names only) that also identify titles. Introduce staff using those titles.
- Highlight one staff member in each quarterly newsletter. This not only

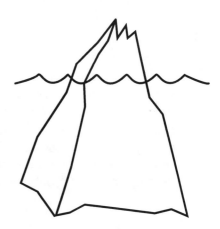

makes the practice seem more real to the clients but also makes the staff member feel more like a member of the team.

- Uniform each team differently, using the same color patterns but in a different style or same style but in different colors, or let the teams tell you what the uniform groupings need to look like (this will allow the power types to emerge).
- Delegate projects not process. Let the staff members determine the group needed to solve a practice challenge. You'll be surprised at the team players who emerge.
- Set team goals and then let the team worry about individual performance. The goal can be gross dollars per day needed to meet the monthly goal. Meeting the monthly goal earns everyone a dinner where you can recognize the star players.
- Make the project of the month (encouraging clients to bring pets in for fecal procedures, heartworm screens, dental procedures, or baths/dips) a contest.
- Remember the bottom-line fact that increased practice revenues are only caused by three factors: (1) more new clients accessing the facility, (2) increased value per unit of contact, and (3) increased number of visits per year per existing client.

THE THREE WAYS TO INCREASE PRACTICE REVENUE

1) More new clients accessing the facility or practice.

2) Increased value per unit of contact.

3) Increased number of visits per year per existing clients.

It is up to the innovative practice leader to find new ways to excite the staff. An excited staff is a staff that will rise to the occasion and excite the clients. Excited clients send in their neighbors or come back in themselves, or both. Excited clients will raise the morale of the staff, which will brighten the practice atmosphere. A cheerier practice atmosphere will excite the veterinarian to become more innovative, and so the cycle will begin to repeat itself ... and profits will follow!

How to Train a Practice Manager

Regarding how to train a practice manager, the first two alternatives that come to mind are "with a whip and a chair" and the more mellow "by example." There are many management theories and a lot of nifty strategies, but the bottom line is that we need results. To get started on the right track, here are a few ideas that have worked in the past:

Step One
Define the job tasks to be done by the practice manager.

Step Two
Determine which responsibilities will be relinquished to the manager and develop the plan for transfer of authority.

Step Three
Develop a list of expected milestones for the new manager and include intermediate objectives needed to meet the goals.

Step Four
Make a list of needed management and leadership skills that the person must possess to accomplish the first three items with only on-site training by existing staff.

The above planning to plan steps are critical. The responsibilities of the new practice manager must include the authority to make unilateral decisions for the good of the practice—decisions that will not be undermined by the practice owner, spouse, or tenured team members. This delegation of authority allows the veterinarian to return to the examination room and client and leave the daily operational concerns to the practice manager.

While there are many management theories, the key one we need to know is what motivates our new practice manager. If we know what the manager's hot buttons are, we can punch them up to accelerate the learning curve. As stated earlier, in the United States, the focus of motivation for healthcare employees has been found to be recognition. This differs from nation to nation, so beware of tips learned in Japan, England, or other foreign countries. An ap-

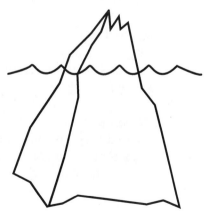

plicant will associate a position with recognition if others perceive the job as important, advancement opportunities are plentiful, personal growth results from the responsibilities, personal effort leads to successful task accomplishment, and successful task accomplishment is rewarded. To be successful, our training and plan for the new practice manager must take into account these motivational factors.

Each practice is unique, and each practice owner has personal preferences for relinquishing authority, but the training must accent the need for group genius. Mere brainstorming with the staff for ideas will never evoke such genius. The most effective managers and leaders understand that tasks are accomplished through the involvement of other people. The staff must become a team, and the team needs to focus on taking moderate risks to become comfortable with innovation. Positive valuing techniques need to be used. Instead of "How do we fix the parking problem?" the team asks, "How do we best improve the parking system?" They need to focus on "what if ...?" and extend beyond customary limitations, ultimately projecting how things need to be in five years. The objectives and goals used to reach the vision must be based on a team consensus, and the practice manager is critical to that process. If you are not yet willing to use a practice manager in that role, you really don't want a true practice manager; rather, you want an extension of your control—a gofer (someone to go-fer-this and go-fer-that).

Team achievement skills are critical. You cannot deliver quality healthcare unless the whole team is involved. Team achievement will result in improved productivity, but there will be many other changes, best measured in qualitative terms such as quality of work life and morale, which also have a significant bottom-line impact. People will enjoy their work more, absenteeism and tardiness will decrease, and the leader will become an approachable colleague rather than a threat.

The areas that need attention in most practices are those in the hospital administrator's sphere of influence.

Time management

Very few practices really know how much time is spent doing which functions. A new practice manager can become an expert in this area in a very short time.

Cost centers

Determining the total cost of individual functions (including equipment replacement) has generally not been done for each outpatient, inpatient, surgical, dental, and ancillary service.

Income centers

Integration of time management results and cost center evaluations will identify income (+/ profit) centers that can be identified for marketing efforts. This integration of information is a natural task for the concerned practice manager who understands personal efforts result in savings or income that offset the manager's new salary.

Performance evaluations

Transferring the 90-day coaching sessions to the practice manager allows for specifically tailored goal setting with staff members to meet the practice goals and augment the group genius efforts.

Inventory management

This will be one of the professional aspects of the practice manager's job. It is estimated that one in five of all employees will likely borrow from the practice sometime without permission. This role will add to the internal control of inventory as well as the cost-effectiveness.

Practice personality

Body language, phone communications, client relations, and intrastaff relationships need to convey concerned care, patient advocacy, and continuity of care. The practice manager can be responsible for the smiles and fun that should permeate the practice.

The bookkeeping, accounts receivable, billing, chart of accounts, POMR quality assurance, and a host of other functions should be transferred once the practice manager earns the team trust and respect. Do not overwhelm a new manager. The job is complex, and the training needs to be a repetitive step-by-step procedure. The manager's job description will never suffice to explain the multiple interrelationships of a veterinary practice. Be patient and have fun.

Look to the Leaders

The best executive is the one who has the sense enough to pick good people to do what needs to be done, and self-restraint enough to keep from meddling with them while they do it.
—Theodore Roosevelt

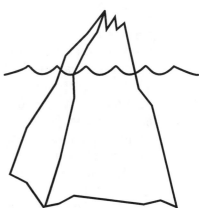

In the leadership of a veterinary practice we need managers as well as leaders. As the old adage goes, "You can lead a horse to water but ..."; no one has ever said, "You can manage a horse to water but ..." In a quality veterinary healthcare delivery system, the leadership is the responsibility of the hospital director while the day-to-day efficiencies are the concern of the practice manager. However, a practice manager must have some specific leadership skills for practice harmony.

Veterinarians are procedure heavy and innovation light, and as the veterinarian goes, so does the practice. In fact, remember that horse you can lead to water but ...? Well, most veterinarians will just stomach tube the beast and get on with life—the heck with waiting! As veterinarians, we have been taught that redundancy provides some degree of safety and protection from disasters in healthcare; our first question is always "What is the reference for that?" We strive to control a disease process, to establish a routine preventive care program, or even to control a set of medical symptoms. In management of the practice's human resources, the routine "control" approach reduces innovation, even though innovation is often needed to save expenses or react to change.

One thing is certain. Progressive veterinary healthcare leaders are winners, and winners are not blue sky dreamers. Rather, they are pragmatic people who live by one thought: Try it now. Winning while keeping a comfortable net requires risk, and it is this willingness to take risks that is the essential difference between the leaders in the profession and the followers. Watch for these leadership traits when training a practice manager:

Stretch

Veterinary medical leaders want their people to reach and stretch for goals and to accomplish more than they ever thought possible. To do this, leaders must work harder than anyone in the practice; they must work long, late hours and make personal sacrifices to accomplish superior results. The price of excellence is time, interest, and attention.

Openness

Veterinary leaders also have to create an environment for discussion, openness, disagreement, and even criticism directed at themselves. If leaders can't be open to views that differ from their own, they will probably have only limited success over the long run. What sustains a practice is the recognition that service is built on a bedrock of listening, trust, and respect for the creative potential of every employee. If leaders treat their people like "personnel," they will act like personnel. If they treat staff like human resources and keep them informed, they will respond with greater innovation and increased productivity. The lines of communication must flow both ways. Facts from paper are not the same as facts from people. The reliability of the person presenting the facts is as important as the facts themselves. But no one will tell the leader the solution to any problem before being asked the right questions. In an atmosphere openness, there must also be truth. Leaders cannot afford to lie. If they do, they diminish the trust others have in them. Even more subtly, leaders lessen their trust in others; they even begin to question their willingness to tell the truth.

Strength

No one wants a weak leader. Veterinary medical leaders who act precisely, with clarity and toughness, are often more respected and gain more loyalty than those who are afraid to make difficult and unpopular decisions. Indecision and impulsiveness only breed uncertainty and discourage creativity. Leaders must know when to be consistent and when to make exceptions. Would you order a subordinate to do something with which he or she disagreed? If you do, you assume the responsibility for the decision; the subordinate is no longer part of it. In the end, the important issue is not who is right but what is right.

Caring

Leaders must support their people because people depend on leaders to make the right choices and to do the right things. After all, people do not really working for a leader; they work with the leader for themselves. Through a lifeline and safety net, a leader must give people the security that he or she won't lead them over a cliff or jeopardize their livelihoods. The leader must be willing to share both the risks and rewards of work. The problem in many practices is that they are overmanaged and underled. *In Search of Excellence,* by Tom Peters, tells us that there are only two ways to create superior performance. First, take exceptional care of your clients through superior service and quality healthcare for their pets. Second, continually innovate. There are no alternatives. The number one productivity problem in America is the presence of managers and leaders who are out of touch with both their people and customers.

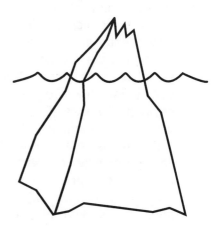

Uncommon Leaders

The greatest strides in human progress have come because of uncommon men and women. We need more uncommon leaders in veterinary medicine, people others can look to when the going gets tough and pressure builds. When we are sick, we don't look for a mediocre physician. If we go to war, we don't seek a mediocre general. And when we send our children to school, we don't desire a mediocre teacher. The same is true for veterinary healthcare.

At the association level—local, state, or national—we have a saying: "Look to the leaders." Look at the leaders in your practice. Are you satisfied with what you see? As Alfred, Lord Tennyson once said, "We are what we are, and if we ever are to be any better, today is the day to begin."

Division of Accountabilities

Table 4.1 is a summary of my beliefs about the basic roles of the hospital director and practice manager. Some have said this list is unbalanced, and that may be so. Life is not always fair, nor is the mantle of leadership; the buck must stop somewhere. My division of responsibilities is based on the mixture needed for effective control within a quality veterinary practice.

Delegation of Control

Neither the hospital director nor the practice manager needs to be overly involved in controlling the day-to-day processes of the trained paraprofessionals. Very few people join veterinary medicine for the money, especially the staff. If the staff are trained properly, how they perform their jobs should be left up to them (within the core values and goals/objectives of the practice). Paraprofessionals need to be empowered to determine their own ways to achieve efficiencies and economies of scale. When someone stumbles during the learning process, remember that only those who attempt to move ahead stumble. Build from the mistake. The key question is "What can *we* do next time to prevent this from recurring?" This is called management by exception.

The delegation of control does not relieve the leadership team, the hospital director and practice manager, from using quality assurance checks. These checks are concerned and caring approaches to the paraprofessional or professional staff, not mandates for reports or feedback. The quality assurance review must be based on a clear line of responsibility between the hospital director and practice manager to keep the team from playing one member of the leadership team against the other.

Regardless of which leader is responsible, the answer lies in the question. An effective question does not insult or intimidate the receiver; it reflects a real concern and a desire to help the staff member succeed. "Why do you ...?" is preferable to "Why don't you ...?" but more effective is "You seem overworked. What can I do to help?"

Table 4.1. Division of responsibilities between the hospital director and practice manager

Functions (Action)	Hospital director (DVM)	Practice manager (non-DVM)	Jointly
Practice philosophy	Primary	Input	
Scope of services	Primary	Input	
Core values	Primary	Input	
Job descriptions	Review	Primary	
Job standards	Review	Primary	
Fiscal goals	Vision		Usually
Break-even analysis	Input	Primary	
Technical procedures	Establish	Update	
Technical efficiencies	Input	Primary	
Technical productivity	Primary	Input	
Salaries	Reserved	Input	
DVM hire/fire	Exclusive		
DVM procedures	Primary	Input	
Staff prehire screen	Standards	Primary w/input	
Staff management		Exclusive	
Staff coaching	Informal	Primary	
Staff problems	Appeals	Primary	
Staff dehire	Input	Primary	
Appraisals	For DVMs	For Staff	
Merit pay	Primary	Input	
Formulary	Exclusive		
Inventory		Exclusive	
Cost of goods sold		Primary	
Internal controls		Primary	
Current ratio		Primary	
Quick ratio		Primary	
Salary as percentage of gross		Primary	
Growth as percentage of increase			Usually
New clients rate		Primary	
Visits/client/year	Primary		
Patient value per year			Usually
Operational team efficacy		Primary	Assesments
Maintenance		Exclusive	
Housekeeping		Exclusive	
Facility expansion			Usually
Marketing		Primary	Niche I.D.
Public relations			Usually

Note: If your veterinary practice is not set up in this manner, the discrepancy is not an issue to debate. The issue is who will do what, when, and why. Use the entire practice team to make your own list!

The Question Is the Answer

Once you become a successful practitioner and build a loyal client base for your practice, you face a dangerous moment in your business career. Will you succeed in transferring the premier practice to another veterinarian, or will you cause it to fall by the wayside and become just another practice? Succeeding requires that you do a strange thing: throw out the knowledge and behaviors that got you where you are and become someone else. If you don't, you are headed for disaster.

In 1989, Dr. G, a very successful practitioner that had built two full-service veterinary practices during his 38 years in the profession, wanted to pass the leadership of the two facilities to four of the six doctors that had worked for him the longest. All the doctors thought they were doing a good job—annual income was approaching a million dollars. "We have a good client-centered practice, a good annual growth in fees, and we promote disease prevention, quality healthcare, as well as responsive sickness care. We are not interested in a low-fee, fast service, high-volume, in-out type practice," stated Dr. G.

But he noticed that the quality, while good, was not what it could be. Nor did client service always live up to its potential. Unless Dr. G could improve and grow, competitors would move into the catchment area. But Dr. G was told by his physician that he needed to take more time off for his personal health, and whenever he returned to a practice, he often found the status quo had not changed. He couldn't get the responses that he had become accustomed to during the last three decades of practice building. He saw waste, inefficiencies, and a loss in the traditional work ethics common in his rural/suburban catchment area. Nobody seemed to want responsibility for fixing the problems. People did only what they were told. How could he get his practices back into gear?

He hired a consultant who told him his expansion dreams were fine and his management plans were well organized but there was a problem.

"The problem is you," the consultant explained. Dr. G was stunned. Him, a problem? Nobody knew the practice, the clients, or the management factors better than Dr. G—he'd built a pair of premier practices from scratch, received accolades from subordinates and colleagues, and was doing far better than any other practice in his area of the state.

"Exactly," said the consultant. "You know everything. You make the decisions. No wonder the other veterinarians don't take responsibility. You won't let them."

As Dr. G listened, he thought of his actions during the past year. He remembered cutting people off, not listening to their opinions, or not letting them make their own management mistakes.

Until now, being the answer man had worked fine for Dr. G. He'd always had the best answers. He'd thought his job was to get his good answers implemented. He now saw that his practices wouldn't catch fire until he got the new owners to supply the answers.

One night, during the consultation, all the veterinarians were sitting around a table, discussing ways to expand the role of the paraprofessional staff in delivering more responsive healthcare. Dr. G. had a great idea about how to make it happen, but then it hit them: "Why the blazes are we doing this? None of us is going to be doing this. We need to get our staff involved in the *how* of the decision process." The consultant had facilitated this discovery, and now Dr. G applied it. Dr. G had to assume the Mike Ditka role of staying off the playing field during practice. He realized that the four new quarterbacks he had identified to take ownership had to lead the team their way.

Dr. G has a new job. He doesn't control practice hours or devise new programs for the veterinarians and staff to pursue. The staff and the four veterinarians who have assumed ownership handle those situations. Dr. G is the coach for the four veterinarians. He is their mentor when needed, but generally, he will be their friend when the pressures make them begin to doubt themselves.

Dr. G has stopped walking through each practice every morning—if he did, he'd be tempted to answer all those questions the staff always have for him. He schedules himself out of most meetings, unless they are restricted to only the four practice owners. His primary question to the owners centers around what is needed to make each practice succeed.

It's not easy relinquishing leadership. The first reaction will usually be wrong. If those owners said, "What do you think about this?" Dr. G needs to ask himself, "Should they be asking me this—or is it their problem? Or is it a challenge for all four new practice leaders to discuss? Or do I need to redefine the problem for them?"

At first, the staff were puzzled at the change in Dr. G's behavior. "We thought he was losing it" was a common concern. But they were told that he was ensuring the two practices and the healthcare delivery teams would fire up and move ahead, just like in the good old days.

Every morning, Dr. G has to remind himself:

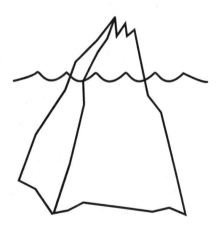

1. The retiring veterinarian's job is to eliminate his or her job—to stop making decisions and to make the right people responsible for the right things.

2. Good people do a good job, dedicated people do a dedicated job, and trained people do a trained job. Untrained people cannot do a good job and lose dedication. In Dr. G's practices, the new owners would have had difficulty being dedicated or good at their jobs without Dr. G becoming a trainer rather than a decision maker.

3. The question is the answer. This statement reminds Dr. G that asking the right question of his people teaches them the skill worth most to the practice: how to think.

4. A retiring leader must change. Before Dr. G attends any meeting, looks at any policy, or responds to any problem, he asks himself, "Is this behavior part of my real job of transferring control and leadership to the new owners?"

5. Look for the good intentions. Always! Before attempting to evaluate why workers make a mistake, look at why they attempted something new and recognize their efforts as a positive influence on the practice. Make this recognition so loud that everyone will hear. The second step, building to a better tomorrow, should be done in private with the individuals who've made the mistakes.

The Moral of the Story

Make staff find the alternatives by asking the leading questions. Do not allow the team members to put their brains in your in box; you won't fill them up anymore while they go play. Ask for two alternatives for solving each problem. Teach them to think; teach them that you value their opinions! If both ideas are okay (that means they "do no harm" to the staff, clients, or practice), let the team members select the one they want to implement and then tell them to keep you informed of their progress.

Good Thinkers Are Made, Not Born!

Never confuse motion with action.

—*Ernest Hemingway*

The effectiveness of thinking is variable. Consider the difference between rapid problem solving and effective long-range planning. It is easy to make a decision in veterinary practice. I see it every day in the practices that I support. The challenge is to make the right decision at the right time.

The Playing Field

The effective thinker is said to have horse sense, common sense, logic, and a philosophy. Definitions reflect that good thinking has little to do with innate intelligence. Most anyone can learn it.

In strategic planning, good thinking depends on SWOT: assessing **s**trength and **w**eakness within the organization and **o**pportunities and **t**hreats external to it. Opportunities and threats must be forecasted 3, 5, and 10 years into the future, and internal strengths and weaknesses must be evaluated to determine how they will affect the pursuit of excellence, profit, and market position in the 3- to 10-year plans.

The reason that most strategic planning efforts fail is that the forecasting has been based on today or the past, not the future. Very common is the tendency to assess the strengths and weaknesses in terms of today's staff and facility rather than after training efforts are completed or after a floor plan changes. "We have never done it that way" is the rule. There are even states trying to remove veterinarians from their existing state board just because they have aligned with Corporate Veterinary Medicine (capitalized to emphasize the fear evoked by this noun). Even if we ignore corporate trends, they will still continue. Smart thinkers decide how to get opponents to work with them. The smart thinkers know that strategic assessment, monitoring change and grabbing opportunity before it passes, is the best tool for meeting the demands of the veterinary marketplace.

Pattern Changing

In today's marketplace, innovation and creativity are needed. Catanzaro & Associates offers three different dental programs to practitioners to inspire them to develop their own plans. A behavior management program is offered that includes an easy to use house-training poster to send home after the first vaccination and information about a puppy club or kitten carrier club. The program integrates receptionist identification of potential needs with technician action for "temporary assistance" while the client and pet visit for an appointment, and it includes an exam room behavior management appointment as an additional benefit to the "easy access" elements of the program. Catanzaro & Associates also offers a geriatric program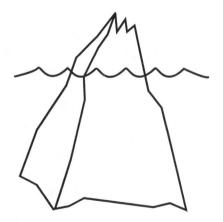

that is started in a way that will persuade the client of its importance: a cardiac screen is done if there is a murmur, or an arthritis assessment is scheduled for the fall, when arthritis is more noticeable. The critical thinker targets what the other person believes is a benefit and starts at that point when trying to make improvements.

Change is harder to accept than improvements. Improvements are in fact changes, but they are less threatening since we have to consider needs before improvements can be made. Reminder cards were an improvement, and sending a series of three was an improvement over sending only one. The way the card makers assisted the acceptance was to offer the benefits in their ads: "A single reminder card brings in 40 percent of your clients, and a series of three brings in over 60 percent." Since very few practices knew their own return rates, these numbers sounded impressive. In fact, the simple addition of a fecal bag (already labeled for the pet) to the first reminder mailing has increased some practices' income significantly. However, the common response to this idea is "we send postcards—we couldn't use that system" (as if the extra 10¢ that an envelope costs and the pennies the fecal bag costs were not offset by the additional fecal sample income). Fuzzy thinking does exist in veterinary medicine.

If you want to encourage someone to make an improvement, offer three of its benefits before suggesting it. For instance, consider how an average companion animal practice doctor would respond to these three questions:

- If I could show you a way to get a routine three-day weekend, would you be interested?
- If I could increase your personal productivity without adding any extra hours to your week, would you want to hear what we could do?
- Would you like to hear about a method that would make most of your clients perceive extra benefits from existing practice programs?

You want to hear the answer, don't you? You expect it will require some form of change, but you *want* to hear the alternatives! I have your attention because I stated the benefits before I suggested evening hours and four 12-hour days for a two-veterinarian practice, M-Tu-W-Th and W-Th-F-Sa (heavy surgery on Wednesday and Thursday, with Isoflurane to extend the available cutting time). There are other schedules Catanzaro & Associates had used with equal success, such as planning a two-week cycle (rather than one-week cycles) for two doctors (on two days, off one, on three days, off one, on four days, then off three), with one week out-of-phase so that the three-day weekends alternate between doctors. Unique thinking leads to revolutionary ideas.

Status Quo

Stasis means death, but many practice owners strive for stasis and consider no change safe. Look back 20 years in your own career development and community leader evolution. The world has changed and so have you. It may have been painful, but it occurred, and you are still enjoying life (at least more than those in a pine box six feet under a headstone). You've probably found the best planning takes time. Snap decisions are generally not the result of thinking but of knee-jerk reactions.

Planning is a process, and it can be taught (see Vol. 1, Chapter Four, "Leadership Skills for Veterinary Practices"). It starts with a clear statement of the problem or task, then moves to an assessment of the potential resources available. This is followed by developing multiple alternatives and assessing the best plan and backup plan (plus an alternate in case the backup plan ends in disaster). The best plan is written, with expected measurements of success clearly defined, and then the accountability for outcomes is described in detail *before* the plan is implemented. The evaluation of this plan is based on how well its implementation meets the criteria for success defined in the plan; the knowledge and experience gained starts a new cycle of planning. This planning process will usually provide a faster result than trial and error, although the start-up (program initiation) is often four times slower. When based on the team's critical thinking, the results are generally more profitable to the practice.

Changing a thinking pattern means challenging the status quo. This is dangerous. It requires using all the resources available, every brain in the practice. It means the receptionists need to talk about client perceptions and the technicians need to be free to talk about traffic flow and sequencing of workload. Each member of the staff must learn that offering input is not dangerous, that everyone's ideas and perceptions are valid and need to be shared. This is the reason good consultants stay in business (good consultants have learned to listen). It is also the reason some consultations will not work (some owners are not willing to listen or change).

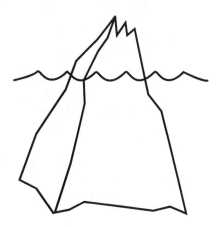

To make the boss listen and expect input from practice staff, someone must train the team members to state the benefits of an improvement before telling the boss the improvement needed. The leader must be willing to accept that no one on staff wants to harm the practice, that staff members only offer opinions because they care and think they may help.

As stated in the great management reference, *Managing from the Heart* (see "Suggested Reading," Vol. 1), the good leader hears with a caring heart, just as the good staff member offers ideas with a caring heart. When members on the team disagree, they don't try to make the other person wrong. Team members acknowledge the greatness in each person, they look for the positive intentions, and they share the truth with compassion. If the leader cannot see the caring in the idea or suggestion, then he or she is generally not looking hard enough. The successful practice leader must be willing to let go of the tree trunk and go out on a limb occasionally ... that is where the apples are!

The Well-Oiled Team

Since the beginning of time, people have joined groups for support and protection. The new middle manager who forgets this basic human need is doomed to fail. The practice with gossipy and snide conversations, or the phrase "That's not my job" being repeated often, has already started on the road to problems. Or staff members' faces are blank or sullen, their voices lifeless and even whiny at times; turnover and absenteeism are higher than expected. Clients are seen as interruptions rather than the most important part of the practice.

People join a group for psychological and material rewards. The more the group satisfies these needs, the more powerful and productive will be the team. People become a team for a combination of five basic reasons:

Recognition

This is the number one motivator in American healthcare delivery teams, even more important than fiscal rewards. The positive feedback of the primary provider is critical, as is the middle manager's appreciation of the staff. Often, community recognition of the veterinary practice will further fulfill this need for recognition.

Belonging

This is the number one motivator in healthcare teams in Europe and Japan and runs a close second in the United States. The identification with a reputable veterinary practice that effectively serves the community satisfies the need for recognition and belonging.

Security

This means the workplace is safe and is an environment where the individual feels cared for by the leadership. Security provides a feeling of family, a common goal, a shared mission in life.

Pride

This is the secret to continuous quality improvement (CQI)—sharing in group achievements by contributing personally. When pride is the work input (this can be sensed by the middle manager), clients will perceive it and consider the practice one of quality; everyone wins!

Individuality

This includes the characteristics and needs of each individual. These must be recognized as well as the resources individuals contribute to the group. A good practice manager relies on and supports the strengths of each person and uses these traits to make the team stronger.

Money is usually one of the top six motivators in healthcare surveys but has never been one the top three reasons for staying with a healthcare delivery team. Successful managers know how to create and nurture individuals and groups. They are the sowers of pride and the harvesters of the quality yields that result.

THE MILLION DOLLAR PRACTICE—A RECIPE FOR SUCCESS

In a unique vision container, stirred with a sacrifice and risk mixer, blend one part cost control and one part financial policy with two parts of market share and one part of client selection. Mix gently with two dashes of diversification and pinch of nonoperating income and let set. Serve with a commitment to the staff, garnished with leadership by example which fits the decor of the serving environment.

Practices Are Not Created Equal

And He said unto them, "All veterinary facilities are not created equal." The waters parted, and the practitioners began to yell. How dare He say their practices were not as good as someone else's! The fact that one out of every two veterinarians graduated in the bottom half of his or her veterinary class, or scored in the bottom half of the boards, does not matter. However, certain things do

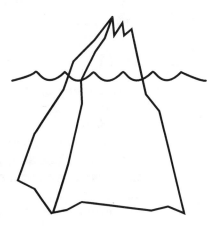

matter. For instance, with pricing strategies, when market leaders charge premium prices, they generally improve their net liquidity. But when practices with a low market share try to charge premium prices, they are entering a dangerous strategy zone. Market leaders often have a better reputation or an image of higher quality that permits them to successfully charge a higher price. Distinguishing between gross and net prices is especially critical in the healthcare professions, where clients may pay different prices for what they perceive are the same services.

Train Your Trainers

The Who

Practice management means change, and change means resistance. The best method to overcome resistance is to provide training to reduce concerns about the unknown. The most effective training method is to train only those key people who are willing to lead others. The best receptionist, the senior technician, and the business manager will be the key people to train your staff (and junior professional staff). Training can be coaching, self-instruction, or on-the-job experience. Regardless of the type, lead time is critical. If done during training, forecasting problems and alternatives provides options. When options aren't discussed until a crisis, staff stress increases and often decisions are less than optimum. And if you don't have time to do the training, you do not understand employee motivation and modern productivity principles.

Being recognized as a trainer can be a significant motivator or, if handled poorly, can cause great disruption. The trainers are staff members hired to be leaders or those members with that natural leadership quality of having followers among your staff. If you bring an outsider into your facility as a trainer, be careful that person doesn't alienate your staff by not knowing your internal processes or procedures.

The What

Areas where trainers can be effectively used to institute change include

Client relations

This is an art and as such requires practice, which usually involves trial and error. Buy pizza and soda and pay overtime wages so that staff can practice phone techniques in role-playing positions. They will get in the swing of it and enjoy the experience, and it will help the recall program when applied. Have the leader for this exercise experience client relations training at a local human healthcare hospital. Such training is commonplace and often learned through autotutorials.

Patient advocacy

This is more than simply caring about the health and welfare of animals. We must express our professional opinions about pets clearly and distinctly. Again, monitor the message as well as the handling of the client's response. Do you tell the owner what the animal "needs," or do you use "should" and "recommend" as if good healthcare was optional? Do you allow the client to waive proper healthcare, or do you try to get a layperson to approve it? Patient advocacy training enables leaders to widen the scope of services if necessary, to use dialogue that includes "need" and "waiver" in client discussions, and to consider most of the human-companion animal bond factors that the Delta Society has advocated for years. If you have not joined the Delta Society, call and tell it you are long past due for this awakening. Its newsletter is excellent for increasing sensitivity and bonding in staff and clients.

Grief/stress counseling

This is another area that requires practice. There are several references on the subject, but discussing grief or stress counseling with a trainer, rather than providing written theory, will provide the methods for communication.

Computer use and literacy

Garbage in—garbage out (GIGO) is the rule. Only when the staff accept responsibility for their computer input will their efforts result in profit. The internal leadership in each work center area can assist in motivating staff members. Pay for a course for internal leaders in which they can learn about computers and software. The investment will be well worth it.

If you analyze how successful business leaders have gotten great results from their staffs, it will become evident that there is nothing intrinsically magic in their methods. They have learned to become sensitive to methods of exciting the employee to believe in what he or she is doing. The basic strategies can be applied to the veterinary practice when they support the philosophy of the practice and scope of services offered. They include

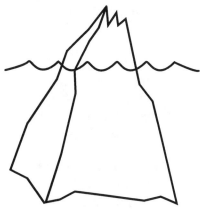

Setting the example

Do you work efficiently? Set deadlines? Prioritize your duties? Do you anticipate problems or try to correct them once they're a threat? You can encourage these skills in your staff by developing them in your practice leadership style.

Giving clear, precise direction

Hasty, unclear, sweeping instructions result in sloppy, unsure, incomplete work. The time you spend thinking about clearly providing a task and explaining it to your staff is time saved in correcting mistakes.

Setting milestones

Work gets done more quickly when a timeline is established. It is best to allow employees' input to determine which part of the project can be done by when. This allows everyone to agree upon and understand the expectations for the project.

Maintaining priorities

Let the staff know which projects are most important to you and which should receive the most time and attention. Keep your staff updated as priorities change.

Delegating responsibility

People work harder and more effectively when they share responsibility for the final product. Besides freeing up your time for other projects, delegating this way develops your staff's judgment in setting priorities and solving problems. They work faster and interrupt you less with problems that previously needed your attention.

Leaving staff members alone to do their jobs

Respect your staff's time. One of the biggest time wasters for most staff members is the boss. Don't constantly interrupt them with unimportant matters or keep them waiting for meetings or instructions.

Encouraging feedback

Staff members should be able to come to you for help. On the other hand, if a staff member finds a quicker or more effective way to do a task, he or she should feel that you are willing to consider a new approach.

Rewarding effort as well as achievement

A staff member who feels appreciated will be encouraged to keep improving. You can offer incentives for good work, such as pay raises, but a sincere thank-you or an accolade along the way can be inspirational. These unexpected rewards cause staff members to strive to fulfill their potential.

The above eight factors are not all-inclusive, nor do they apply equally to all management styles and veterinary practices, but they are the basis for success in any small business operation. Veterinary medicine has become a true small business, with competitors in close proximity. The human resources within any practice need to be considered as a fixed expense, but they are also the only real variable we have left that can affect the profit bottom line of a practice. Within the comfort zone of the practice owners, the above factors can be used to find and empower trainers to implement and achieve success in a more effective and efficient management approach.

The Why

Developing trainers from within your staff is actually a form of delegation of authority as well as responsibility. Such delegation allows the veterinarian to increase client/patient time and profit. By encouraging self-supervision within work center staff, delegation ensures the administration's directions are carried out. Recognizing trainers also provides a way to help acknowledge employees for their efforts and expertise. Image is a primary motivator in healthcare delivery, and whenever we can give someone a title or a specific area of responsibility for acknowledgment and recognition, then we have added leverage to our motivation program.

Orchestrating a team effort takes practice, and it cannot come from the top only. In the best case, all participate and contribute, but in most practices, key people must carry the momentum. By identifying those trainers, we develop their natural leadership abilities and capitalize on their energies.

The Bottom Line

Having multiple trainers means changes can be initiated on multiple levels at one time. The dynamic nature of the veterinary practice requires decisions be made by all work centers for maximum market impact and client response.

Training your trainers is fun and builds harmony and feedback. It makes policies and procedures yield to common sense,

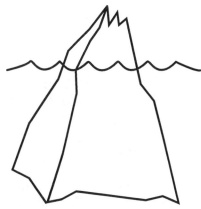

which increases efficiency. And better efficiency and harmony yield improved net.

Train Dogs; Nurture People

A brain is a terrible thing to waste. To get veterinary practices to invest in *every* staff member's development on a recurring basis is a perpetual challenge. Usually a new employee is assigned a title, graded on a scale from 1 to 10 (1 being at the low end), and chastised for any mistakes. Some consultants even advise that if the staff member is below an eight, that person needs to be fired.

Learning for Life

A person is the sum of his or her life experiences, education, and environment. Each person brings a unique set of values, ethics, and attitudes to a veterinary healthcare delivery team. This team has been formed by a veterinarian with his or her own set of values, ethics, and attitudes. For years we have talked about training. I have, also. But in many cases, something has been lacking in the tasking.

First, I thought the problem resulted from veterinary education being so process oriented, with step-by-step procedures for everything from orthopedics to floating fecal matter. Then I thought it was the result of the paradigms of our education system, where everyone is graded on a five-point scale. Eventually I evolved the concept that veterinary practitioners feel they are so busy they don't have time to educate their staff. Self-education is more common than practice training schedules.

We hire people for their strengths, yet we target their weaknesses during the appraisal process. American industry spent over $18 billion in 1994 on training. Most of the current literature on training takes a step-by-step form: "Ten ways to ...," "Twelve keys to ...," or "The critical steps to ..." Sounds a lot like canine obedience training to me. Now corporations want training information on videocassettes, audiocassette tapes, software, or other electronic media. Maybe this is so we don't have to be involved in the learning process. But helping staff members apply what they learn to previous life experiences, personal attitudes, and the current environment is what enables them to become practice team members.

No Fear

A trainer must be a mentor, finding each person's strengths and building on them. The veterinary staff are the first and last contact for clients, many of whom are stressed because they don't know what is wrong with their pets, what will happen, or what it will cost. Staff members must be confident about how to apply what they know. Their training must develop this trait.

The most common form of training is lightning bolt education, from which staff learn what they shouldn't do. Their training is based on the wrath of the managers. Negative reinforcement is like dog obedience training with a pinch collar. But dogs do not have to be trained with this collar; a better one has been developed. The newer style collars provide instinctive pressure, and the dog responds to positive reinforcement within minutes. The response can be duplicated by any family member at the end of the leash. Appropriate behavior is reinforced with accolades. So it is with the nurturing process. A practice manager must be a practice leader and accomplish objectives through the staff working toward a common outcome. A manager works with projects and costs while a leader works with people who have feelings, and feelings are nurtured, not taught.

A leader partners a staff member with sources, peers, and clients. This triad is the key to successful staff development. The sources are emerging software programs, the new American Veterinary Medical Association staff texts (Crisp books), and the abundance of texts and short courses available in every locality. The peers are the healthcare team members, from the doctor to the technician to the receptionist to the animal caretaker. This group must discuss, debate, and implement a plan for concerned care that includes the patient, the client, the staff quality of life, and the practice liquidity. The clients are the best partners for staff development because they are the ones accessing the services. The staff member who listens, who determines what clients want and can get it to them, and who gets clients back for the next visit is the successful student. The ones who make excuses, compare needs to policies, or follow the process to the letter are the ones who stifle success.

Tailored Training

Like human history, training has had many eras. In the Neanderthal practice, you trained yourself by watching the person next to you. This was called trial and error. In the Cro-Magnon practice, the staff member who knew a process best trained all the others, no matter how tedious the process or whether or not it improved practice productivity. This resulted in the caveat "we have always done it this way." In the

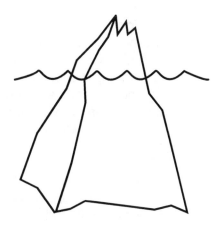

Industrial Age practice, training was the machine. People entered the room, 100 slides of knowledge were dumped into every head simultaneously, and the people departed, properly illuminated. The gimmick-of-the-moment club. In the Modern Era practice, people receive systematic introductions to the practice and the total environment. They are allowed to develop skills and confidence. Then they are made accountable for specific outcomes that they have developed, which creates pride in their evolution. They are expected to make continuous quality improvements to meet client, peer, and practice needs, which nurtures personal ownership in job skills and career development.

The concepts of the Modern Era practice are not easy for most practices to implement. It takes time and commitment to nurture each person. But there are a few methods the caring leaders can use to do this:

Triage training
The old paradigm was one-size-fits-all training. The caring leader prescreens procedures for those that will build upon the new staff member's strengths. Remember, the reasons the employee was hired. Once early wins are achieved, the more difficult desired outcomes are addressed, in a protracted and planned training cycle, so small-step successes are possible on the way to the major accomplishment.

Reality training
Addressing the problems of the practice is important, but addressing the problems perceived by the learner is more critical to success. A leader must be aware of the virtual reality of a veterinary practice: the client sees something different from the doctor, and the staff something different from the client or doctor. Unless all perceptions are addressed by a mentor close at hand, a new staff member will make wrong assumptions.

Redesign
The best method for nurturing staff is to redesign the jobs and tasks around the strengths of the people available and the client demands. At some point, the less desirable tasks must be allocated, but when building upon strengths, the honey comes first, so the bitter is more palatable. The leader who cares enough to build on the strengths of the individual worker will bond staff and clients to the practice.

T.L.C.
Tender loving care, not thin layer chromatography, is required for nurturing team members. Constructive criticism is a negative—period! Knowing what underlies someone's attitude means knowing what is

happening to him or her outside the practice. It is caring about that staff member as a person. Caring is a positive. *No one cares how much you know until they know how much you care.*

Leadership is critical to training. A great trainer is someone who can regularly communicate in terms that a staff member can comprehend, someone who can talk without buzzwords, who understands the learner's point of view. Learning happens most often and best in practices where the leadership signals early on that learning is what the organization is all about, and training is not done for just the continuing education hours accumulated. An example of good practice leadership is one that requires *one* new idea implemented for each funded day of CE, for *any* doctor or team member of the practice attending *any* course. Leaders that expect an idea to be implemented without having to give approval show a high degree of trust in the capabilities of the team member.

Leaders who develop their empathy and imagination to sense training needs also create some of the situations to allow the team to see the needs also. Using this method of "practice discovery" allows the leader to respond to the needs of the team. Using the team brain power to devise a method or alternatives to address the "discovered" need allows development of a custom training program that the staff has already bought into during the discovery. Seeing the problems and challenges through the eyes of others is the key to training success. Wherever the staff is thinking, that is where the training needs to be.

Overcoming Obstacles

Obstacles—those frightful things we see when
we take our eyes off our goals.
—Dr. T. E. Cat

Some practitioners erroneously believe that solving immediate practice management problems is the best way to change productivity and performance. A better approach is to cultivate ideas whose application and impact range beyond the task of the moment. To overcome inertia and get things done, you must rely on breakthrough and follow-through skills.

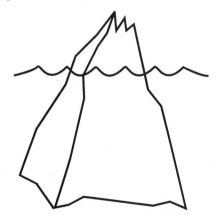

Breakthrough Skills

As a team leader or a team member, you must first learn how to present your ideas in a comprehensive and enlightening manner:

Cover your bases
Before you show off your personal planning skills, make sure you are seen as doing a good job with your current responsibilities. If you don't have time to think beyond the immediate concerns on most practice days, delegate the more repetitive day-to-day responsibilities to dependable staff members.

Network
Before you suggest an idea at a team meeting, try to get a feel for the other team members' interests and concerns. Know the problems they face and the solutions they have developed and address the issue at hand in terms that include their interests.

Seek opportunities
View problems as opportunities to solve challenges. A strategic thinker sees multiple alternatives in events that others view as crises or failures. Nurture this attitude within the practice team.

Be positive
Make your suggestions in a nonconfrontational way. If your idea impacts others, soften your approach with phrases like "What are your thoughts on ...?" Remember, the staff within almost every practice care and want to help. Their suggestions almost always come with good intentions. Look for the caring intention *before* you evaluate their suggestions.

Don't limit yourself
Do not hesitate to make suggestions that are not related to the bottom line. Clients must believe you care before they believe in your healthcare plan. The value of an idea to a practice is measured in quality of life as well as quality of care. Practice benefits can and should go beyond saving money or producing profit.

Follow-through Skills

Planning a project can be completely different from implementing it and far more difficult than ever anticipated. When projects stall, everyone becomes frustrated. Projects stall for many reasons, but the obstacles that block projects' completion have some common features. The first secret to proactively enhance the follow-through is to recognize obstacles of your own making:

Fantasies

You can envision how well a plan will work and are far happier doing this than overseeing the actual implementation hassles. You need to set the fantasy aside and get your hands dirty. Edison had a vision of how a lightbulb should work but had to build over 1,000 of them to turn his vision into reality. Are you ready for 999 failures before becoming famous for your new ideas within the professional or client community?

Fear of failure

Fear that results will fall short often causes us to let a project quietly die rather than live with poor results. Remind yourself that concrete results, even those that fall short of expectations, are far better than none at all.

Invisible ruts

A common pitfall is mindlessly following old habit patterns. We have learned from what we've done, and know what works, but a practice plateau or lifestyle stagnation is caused by nonchange rather than the pursuit of unique or new experiences. Ask if those old stale protocols are important, and if your tendency is to retain them, determine why. If the why is simply "We have always done it this way," then bypass the protocols and get things done.

Comforting mythologies

Don't fall prey to the slogans or comforts of tradition. Southern California community needs are different from those of the rest of the United States; suburban needs are different from those of small town rural America. Marketing gimmicks must be tailored to the community needs; they must not be taken from some article or consultant who has not even been in your practice. If you believe everything is fine as long as everybody is busy, you might overlook the benefits of new projects.

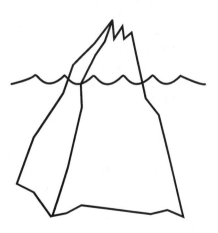

Egotism

Thinking that your own intuition and insights are infallible cuts you off from your colleagues' ideas. Doctor, paraprofessional, or animal caretaker, it does not matter. Everyone has a mind, and each mind has unique ideas. Objectively review all suggestions, including your own, and implement the best.

Failure to delegate

You may be shouldering the whole burden because nobody else is as effective as you are—or because you don't want to share the credit when a project is done. Either way, you place the project at risk. Your odds of success increase greatly when you take on only the tasks that best suit your abilities and let others take on the rest. Train each person to a level of trust, then delegate the accountability for the outcome to him or her (not just the process). Let each person improve the program.

Inflexibility

When an approach is not working, substitute something more positive. If your staff do not implement your ideas, ask them for alternatives. Let them develop unilateral plans and put those into action, then evaluate them at 90 days for benefits. Never veto ideas just because they are not yours! Flexibility often requires taking a step backward, but it ends up being more productive.

Love of intrigue

They are either with you or against you, right? Put aside petty intrigues and enlist everyone's help. A them-versus-us practice staff will never be a healthcare team. Only "we" can create harmony and success. If you love intrigue more than progress, or you prefer to take credit and give blame rather than take blame and give credit, go into politics or the spy business.

Power up for Problem Solving

In our daily routines we rely upon habits to get jobs done, but when we need a creative or innovative solution, we often don't know where to start. There are tools that teach creative problem solving. They don't give you genius; they simply pull out the genius within you. For those practices that do not have computers, or have computers that are not user-friendly, the softcover text *A Kick in the Seat of the Pants or A Whack on the Side of the Head,* by Roger von Oech, provides exercises, stories, tips, and techniques to help you strengthen each of your creative skills. The books are sold separately, but sometimes you can find them together with a deck of innovation cards, and the set is called a "Whack Pack." These aids can be used to awaken creative skills in your staff, since the staff are the best problem solvers you have. Then all you have to do is capture the great ideas from the flow of innovation.

For those who are computer friendly, or at least acquainted, new software programs that enhance creativity, innovation, and problem-solving abilities come out every week. It is smart to stop at the local software store and discuss your needs with a hacker on the staff. Do not buy a software product until you have booted it up yourself, fed in a current problem or idea, and determined what the program can do for you. These programs are just logic trees that can be used by most decision makers who want assistance in innovative and creative thinking. Not all programmers have the same logic tree as you, and very few understand healthcare delivery, much less veterinary medicine.

Doing Gets It Done

When a project stalls, making a new beginning can provide the spark that lets the project catch fire. Inactivity leads to inertia; often a consultant must be called in to break the paradigms that formed the inertia. Picture your practice as a giant boulder resting on a level playing field. Time has caused it to settle into a depression. The boulder can only be moved an inch or two, and if something isn't immediately added to the depression, the boulder will return to where it was. If an idea rock is added to the void created by moving the boulder, it will not be able to return to the old position. Each movement of the boulder allows another idea rock to be added to the temporary void. In time, the depression will be filled with rocks, and the boulder will be moved on the level playing field in the desired direction with a lot less effort than ever before.

When searching for breakthrough or follow-through ideas, use your natural logic for a five-minute boulder-moving effort. If you are stuck, decide that you will start to work on a task at a particular time and will continue for five minutes. At the end of the five minutes, determine if you want to continue another five. Make the same determination again, and so forth. This enables you to take focused action rather than view the project as a behemoth.

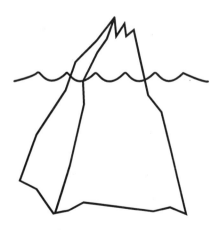

If all else fails, stop, relax, and remember the words of Isaac Newton: "If I have ever made any valuable discoveries, it has been owing more to patient attention than to any other talent."

Application Exercise

As stated in the Introduction, mind mapping is an excellent technique not only for generating ideas but also for developing intuitive capabilities. Use the iceberg ideas you have added on the odd-numbered pages and the concepts you have drawn from this chapter to expand the following mind map.

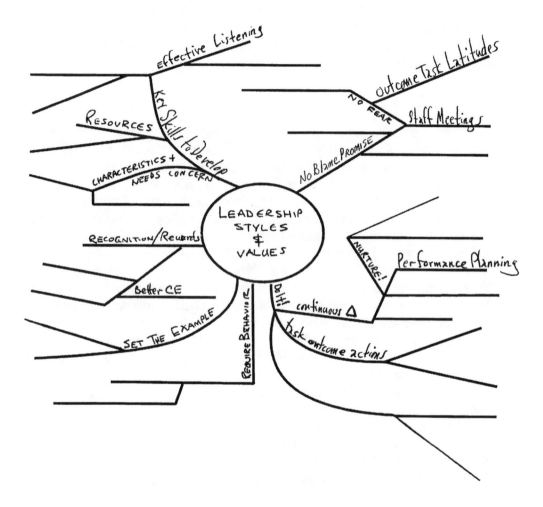

CHAPTER FIVE

Building the Learning Environment

Innovation and creativity must be relearned after
school is over.

The major problem in veterinary medicine is that we are a young profession, and we are defining the business as we go. The first companion
animal hospital was built in 1929, and the American Animal Hospital
Association was not even started until 1938—this means most all practice
owners learned from some guy who was in a farm practice and decided to
see the smaller companion critters—that is why we call it "small animal
medicine." Look at the following habits and traditions, and the alternatives,
and you may start to understand.

■ We have routinely scheduled one doctor in one room with a single column of clients, yet physicians use four to six rooms per doctor, and den-
tists are double that number (now think of the old-time veterinarian, in
his truck, visiting one farm at a time).
❏ If you believe in the New American Veterinary Practice, and understand that "staff produces net," review high-density scheduling in Vol.
2 for some alternative methods.

■ We have routinely charged anesthesia by the animal size, yet isoflurane
only costs $6 per hour to use (now think of the value of the cow in the
chute, the veterinarian and his black bag, and the cost per pound to
make her well).
❏ If you want the New American Veterinary Practice, consider this sequence, with each item/procedure deserving its own fair price:

- preanesthetic blood screen (varies with age and physical condition),
- induction (less than $20, but covers most overhead),
- initial maintenance (not by weight, but for 30 minutes minimum),
- continuing anesthesia maintenance (by the minute),
- postsurgery pain medication,
- postsurgery hospitalization,
- then the follow-up plan.

■ We have made preanesthesia blood screening voluntary, IV supportive therapy during surgery an exception, and always say, "But what about the price?"
  ❑ In quality practices, the blood screen is mandatory now.
  ❑ In progressive practices that worry about animal pain and rapid recovery, supportive IV therapy during surgery is mandatory.
  ❑ Pricing is secondary to the need of the patient and the need of the provider in quality care—compromise of professional standards is a liability.

■ We have always charged hospitalization cage and run space by the animal size (almost like a feedlot operation).
  ❑ The value is in the time, process, and people involved, not the kibble in the bowl:
    - od/bid cases—level one hospitalization
    - tid/qid cases—level two hospitalization
    - IV cases—level three hospitalization (also postsurgery)
    - ICU cases—level four hospitalization
  ❑ Yes, this can be used in bandaging (no joint, one joint, two joint, with an appliance or supportive wrap or without) ... start rethinking your habits!

■ We have always been afraid to sell our knowledge and, instead, have routinely sold "things" (e.g., vaccines at major inflation markups, the cost of the "exam" instead of the doctors' consultation).
  ❑ Producer veterinarians have started charging for their time, even on the telephone, with clients.
  ❑ Producer veterinarians have started software computer systems to manage the husbandry for their clients and charge for this service.
  ❑ Producer and farm veterinarians charge by the mile to get to a client, yet specialists who travel between companion animal practices usually do not.
  ❑ When the pendulum swings, why do the companion animal veterinarians always wait for the other guys to change first?

■ We have always managed companion animal practices by expense comparisons, yet the traditional veterinary software has been developed like very fancy cash registers, only tracking income factors (and a mail merge for client mailings).
 ❑ Without expense to income relationships, you cannot determine net!
 ❑ Program-based budgeting (see Vol. 2) provides program and procedure factors for managing practices—the things that make the front door swing!
 ❑ The new veterinary software systems, in 32-bit Windows technology, will track healthcare delivery, in picture and word, and the better systems will also have automatic data download capabilities to existing spreadsheet programs for easy practice use.

Like the new veterinary graduates who can transplant kidneys and do orthopedic surgery like heroes, but have never seen a cat bite abscess, done a dentistry, or even soloed on an OHE, our knowledge is not always calibrated to the level we need it. This requires a supplemental learning opportunity and a new perspective on building a practice-based learning environment. This is the territory of the uncommon leader in the New American Veterinary Practice. Look at the boss types, and you will better understand the challenge ahead.

Some people characterize the boss as a bear or a pussycat, and staff members get titles like lions, tigers, turtles, or other sundry beasts. It can be fun to recognize your coworkers' animal types—and also to identify your own. Of course, no one is the same animal all the time. Stressful situations bring out the beast in us, while harmony elicits a different response.

Working with people is often more demanding than lion taming. Perhaps that's because there is an animal inside many of us, suggest Frances Norwood and Annette Nunez, professors at the University of Southwestern Louisiana. They use animals to describe traits of difficult people and then suggest ways to tame them. I have adapted their work to veterinary medicine to start this chapter:

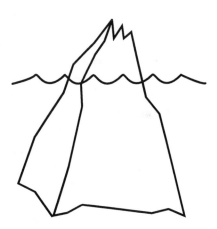

Bulls
They come out charging, attacking the other person, usually because they feel frustrated. Because they feel their victims are inferior, they believe they have tremendous power and often act abusive, abrupt, and intimidating. To manage bulls:

1. Let them speak for a while to let off steam.
2. Sit or stand deliberately and dramatically to get their attention.
3. Call them by name and maintain eye contact.
4. Ask them to have a seat.
5. Present your ideas forcefully.
6. Refuse to argue.
7. Be as friendly as possible.

Snakes

They enjoy blending in with the surroundings and striking suddenly when their victims least expect it. To manage snakes:

1. Bring problems out into the open.
2. Involve the group.
3. Smoke out hidden problems through surveys, suggestion boxes, etc.

Cheetahs

They burst forth in sudden temper displays (a tactic learned early in life to cope with fear and helplessness), as an automatic response to threat. To manage cheetahs:

1. Sincerely try to alleviate their fears.
2. Help them regain confidence and control.
3. Talk with them privately.

Macaw Parrots

They talk and chatter—sometimes sense, sometimes nonsense. They feel powerless and think others should behave in certain ways, and they complain when they don't. To manage macaws:

1. Give them your full attention and maintain eye contact so they'll feel important.
2. If they have a complaint, don't jump to conclusions before you hear the matter out.
3. Ask for facts and get the complaint in writing.

Beavers

They are hardworking and proficient, but they arouse other employees' jealousy and suspicion. They often are underpaid because they don't demand more or are bypassed for promotion to keep them doing their present jobs. To manage beavers:

1. Don't exploit them and don't make them favorites.

2. Advise them to channel some energy into developing better relation-ships with fellow employees.

Cubs

They are humorous, friendly, and cooperative. They agree, whether or not that's what they truly think. Needing to be liked leads them to make unrealistic commitments. To manage cubs:

1. Let them know they can be honest.
2. Compliment them.
3. When you suspect their commitments, say, "I don't think I could do that in the time you've allotted. When I did that it took me more time."
4. Look for true feelings in their humor.

Hyenas

They chill out people's positive feelings. They lack faith in other people and wilt them with sarcasm and doubts. To manage hyenas:

1. When they predict failure, ask: "What's the worst thing that can hap-pen?"
2. Make positive statements about past successes.
3. Show your determination to take action and succeed.

Rhinoceroses

They are strong, knowledgeable people, whose know-it-all attitudes are overbearing. Their ideas are best; yours unimportant, except when they can be used to point out your shortcomings. To manage rhinoceroses:

1. Be certain your facts are correct when you present ideas to them.
2. Repeat what they say to avoid their overexplanations.
3. Use questions when you express dis-agreement.

Peacocks

They pretend to be experts but aren't and so often give wrong or partially correct ad-vice. To manage peacocks:

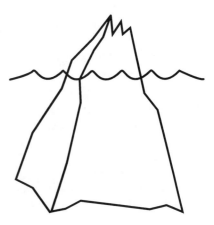

1. Let them maintain their dignity but don't rely on their information.
2. Remind them of facts diplomatically.
3. Give them opportunities to strut their stuff.

Turkeys

They can't make a decision. They're usually nice but hope most situations will resolve themselves or be forgotten before they must decide. To manage turkeys:

1. Talk through the decision-making process step by step.
2. Listen carefully to identify their fears.
3. Slow why ideas or proposals are worthwhile.
4. Emphasize the need to be decisive.

Ostriches

They stick their heads in the sand, handling painful situations in non-committal ways. They tend to avoid committing to other people and themselves during a course. To manage ostriches:

1. Use questions to get them to talk. Don't fill in silences.
2. Summarize what they say, ending the summary with an open-ended sentence.
3. Listen attentively when they talk. End the discussion if they clam up but set up another appointment.[1]

The Learning Practice Environment

To create the learning practice environment, it takes much more than just categorizing the staff. In fact, in a learning environment, evolution will keep the "animals" changing on a daily and weekly basis, and that process is where the New American Veterinary Practice (Vol. 2) leadership really excels. The discipline required for effective leadership takes five forms.

The Five Disciplines

Systems Thinking

- Focuses on the whole, not on the pieces
- Is concerned about patterns and relationships, not isolated events
- Considers role of the person in the practice whole
- Knows symptomatic treatment causes long-term resistance

---

[1]Modified from Frances W. Norwood and Annette V. Nunez, "Managing the Animal within Us," *SAM Advanced Management Journal,* 2331 Victory Parkway, Cincinnati, Ohio 45206, vol. 52, no. 2.

- Is critical as any practice grows past one provider
- Helps fuse the other four disciplines together

Core Values and Vision
- Focuses on what and why
- Negotiates when and how from values
- Helps individual share purpose and destiny of the practice team
- Inspires and connects the process of creation and nurturing

Participative Process in Team Learning
- Believes the whole is smarter than its parts
- Dialogue, not debate!
- Raises the group's collective intelligence and awareness
- Begins when participants suspend their own beliefs and explore other possibilities
- Focuses on the team as the fundamental learning unit

Attitude of Personal Mastery
- Deepens personal vision and physical, spiritual, and emotional strength
- Involves dedication to become the best one can be
- Believes in a continual process of improving the connection between individual and team

Mental Models
- Challenges the deep-rooted assumptions of history
- Believes vision moves group forward, while bias holds it back
- Requires changing the way you think and how you approach challenges
- Strives for flexibility and adaptive change

Even when a leader exercises these five disciplines, some people just don't get it! The challenge often lies in understanding how adults learn and remembering that each situation and each staff member is different (review the situational leadership and effective teaching leadership skills, Vol. 1). It has been shown in many studies that the usable knowledge retention rates of adults vary with the method of education:

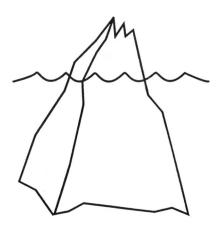

5 percent in lecture

20 percent with questions
50 percent with good case studies
75 percent with on-the-job training (OJT)
95 percent when they must teach it

This is not that difficult a concept if we think about how this text is organized. From the Introduction and Chapter One to this point, this volume has reinforced the importance of

Vision
Clear expectations
Developing skills and knowledge
What leaders can do to make a difference

The vision is the big picture. It is the basis for the mission statement and practice philosophy. Where the usual challenge emerges is that the vision is not based on reproducible core values, and therefore the practice philosophy cannot be an extension of core values. A constantly changing community and veterinary practice environment requires consistent core values so people can make a change without checking with the boss. Keep this example in mind:

In times of calm, we established the new practice ground rules in an open staff meeting. P-R-I-D-E was used to define the core values—Patient needs came first, followed by Respect for the patient and each person (clients, staff, doctors, etc.); Innovation was a personal expectation, while Dedication was a client-service behavior requirement. Excellence was the standard for all actions.

Whenever the "control freak" boss tried to get involved in the middle of a staff member's ongoing project, he would usually start by asking, "Why are you doing that?"; the "one-letter" response (e.g., P or R or I or D or E) was a method to politely tell the boss he was stepping over the boundary again and overcontrolling the change process. It took time, and we had to reinforce the process frequently, but it finally started to work!

Once the vision is established, expectations are developed. These are the practice members' expectations that other members will be

■ Team players
■ Flexible

- Lifelong learners
- Innovative
- Accountable for outcomes
- Patient and client focused

The proper practice environment, a harmonious learning organization, allows the development of skills and knowledge—if we hire for attitude! If you remember to apply the skills for situational leadership and forming the group (Vol. 1), and develop a continuous change environment (see the previous chapters), then you can address the feedback mechanisms used during the development of skills and knowledge (remember "persuading and coaching" during "forming and storming" in Vol. 1). Also please remember: feedback must never be punitive! Use the following as starting points in your own leadership narratives:

"When we ..."	No accusations
"I feel ..."	No blame
"The results appear to be ..."	No value judgments
"Because I ..."	Describe connection
"I would like ..."	Personal preference
"What do you think?"	Listen totally
Pause for discussion response	Let others talk

Mistakes are opportunities to grow and learn!

VISION ➪ Expectation ➪ Skills & Knowledge ➪ What can be done to make a difference

The final stage of the flow, what can be done to make a difference, is often mediated by the doctor's fear of failure. This fear, which does not belong in the New American Veterinary Practice, can be changed. Here is a grading scale system to help assess the real threat caused by the monsters hiding in the closet, the fears so common in every new endeavor.

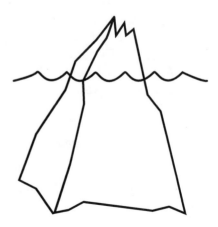

Step One
Make a strength assessment: capability A to D; interest 1 to 4.

Step Two
Ask, "How could we mess this up?": likelihood 1 to 4; impact A to D.

Step Three
Develop success measures: *measurement drives improvement.*

Step Four
Take a weekly pulse by monitoring cost, quality, service, and procedure trends.

Step Five
Ask, "When you were last caught between the rock and the hard place, what happened?" Remember the alternatives we have discussed:

Prevention or change
Clarification of boundaries
Elimination of red tape
Protection of risk takers
Celebration of the learning effort

Finally
Remember the bottom line of the entire practice culture: core values.

The central thing about the central thing is the central thing.

As already discussed, the measurement of success is established at the beginning of a program. It is not that different from any road trip—if we know where we are, and we have a decent map showing the area between here and there, and we know when we need to get to there, then the route can be plotted to incorporate all the parameters, critical and personal, that must be considered during the journey. Sure, there are some control freaks who never stop for family hygiene breaks, but we are talking about a journey of a learning organization—the New American Veterinary Practice!

In veterinary practice, the core values help establish the what and how, but the team and the community establish the who and when. Measurements can be subjective or objective (review the key result areas in Vol. 2). Regardless, they must be known by the staff (e.g., the DIG team, Appendix A) before they implement the system so that they can be flexible and innovative. Just remember the following statement, and you will be okay.

What you choose to measure drives the culture,
and the practice culture drives behavior.
Measurements align and focus the culture!

	Statement—full commitment to true/false response required	Circle One
1.	In times of great change, communication is critical. We need to keep telling people where we are going.	True or False
2.	It is critical to ensure everyone understands why the practice most come before the individual in daily operations.	True or False
3.	It is important that the practice leadership takes care of people and their feelings during times of great change.	True or False
4.	In times of great practice change, people need more emphasis on teamwork and interdependence.	True or False
5.	When changing a practice program, individual characteristics must change before behavior traits can be addressed.	True or False
6.	In times of great change, people need more, not less, feedback on how they and the practice are doing related to the goals.	True or False
7.	For fastest results, the style of leadership required during a change process must be a very democratic and supportive.	True or False
8.	Too much emphasis on learning "new skills" during times of change makes people feel even more insecure.	True or False
9.	For the change process to work effectively, the leader must be willing to meet the team members "halfway" in the alternatives.	True or False

Fig. 5.1. How you deal with change: a test.

The process of change is intertwined with the practice culture. Issues can be defined by outcome (New American Veterinary Practice) or by process (traditional veterinary medicine). In Figure 5.1, there is not a single true statement when viewed from the New American Veterinary Practice perspective. The new culture allows far more flexibility. As an example, look closer at number 1:

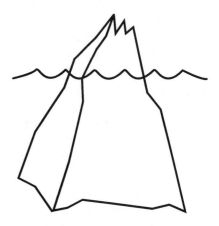

"In times of great change, communication is critical. We need to keep telling people where we are going."

Communication is the getting and giving of information, and telling people something is not participative. The "where we are going" takes the flexibility out of the process, and "keep telling" compounds this problem. Consider number 3:

> "It is important that the practice leadership takes care of people and their feelings during times of great change."

Good leaders are empathetic, but rather than take care of people, they allow people to take care of themselves. Feelings might be addressed, but often these represent resistance, requiring no corrective action except for a release of the person not willing to change.

The nine true-false statements provided do pose a great starting point for leadership-team discussions, and since the practice culture starts with senior management, this simple formula for success must be understood.

$A^2 = G^2$

Always	**A**lways
Do	**G**et
What	What
We've	We've
Always	**A**lways
Done	**G**ot

Since the practice culture starts with senior management, management must address where each person is in the total scheme of things. Not all staff members are ready to soar—in fact, many have a hard time walking and chewing gum. This is most often a result of leadership training, or lack thereof, not staff learning. The Effective Teaching leadership skill (Vol. 1) includes Evaluating (another leadership skill discussed in Vol. 1), and that means there is a constant need to restore balance to keep a group together while accomplishing a task. The cycles of learning and change are illustrated in Figure 5.2.

Regardless of what the leadership thinks, it is the individual staff members who make the difference, and they are not all at the same place at the same time about similar issues. Most staff start in the lower left quadrant (which represents the forming stage of Group Development, another leadership skill discussed in Vol. 1) and progress into the upper left-hand quadrant (which represents the storming stage of Group Development). It is here that the stages of resistance become most visible.

First stage of resistance (dumb and happy) = excuses
• People need readiness to learn—not just training.
• "What's in it for them" is needed.

Clued In & Uncomfortable	**Awkward but Trying**
Feel: know what you don't know	Feel: aware of the learning process nervous about mistakes
Show: aware and awkward	Show: tentative/cautious optimism glimmers of hope
Need: persuading & coaching characteristics and needs understood by leader mastery of the basics understanding of the practice plan reflection opportunities for group and person	Need: set-the-example leaders "How to" stuff chance to represent the group practice, practice, practice feedback & mentoring
Clueless & Comfortable	**Proud & Accomplished**
Feel: don't know what you don't know skeptical	Feel: sure and secure positive and creative
Show: complacency, "ho hum" always done it that way	Show: pride & achievement independence
Need: a discovery rationale for learning clear directions detailed instructions	Need: reinforcement by consult OK for letting go of old ways opportunities for innovation

Fig. 5.2. Stages of learning and change.

Second stage of resistance ("I told you so") = fear of failure
- People need the opportunity to make mistakes.
- Celebrate the attempt.
- "What can we do better next time?" is the question.

Staff who reach the upper right quadrant (the norming stage of Group Development) facilitate delegation, while those in the lower right quadrant (the performing stage of Group Development) allow the leadership to join in and start to enjoy the learning organization. But as pointed out in Vol. 1, nothing is forever. A new person on the team, or a new project, will cause the cycle of learning and change to start all over again. When seeking the best for your practice, use the following questions to help you better understand where each team member is in the cycle.

1. What images come to mind when you think of a healthy future?

2. What is the role of veterinary healthcare in your community?

3. What excites you about this direction?

4. What roles, jobs, and/or responsibilities exist for veterinary healthcare professionals?

5. How do you see yourself fitting into this new image?

6. What are the emerging roles for veterinary extenders?

7. What are the things you need to do to move toward the new image (direction)?

8. What has held you back? What holds you back now?

9. What are the first steps you can take (e.g., training, networking, affiliating, etc.)?

Know What You Don't Need to Know

*Leadership control is a function of well-defined outcomes and
setting parameters on the latitude for resource use; it is getting things
done through other people.*
—Dr. T. E. Cat

As a practice grows, so does the number of things or people who need management attention. If the veterinarian attempts to be in all places at every crisis, the practice of healthcare delivery suffers. If the veterinarian abdicates the crisis solution process, healthcare delivery suffers—but there are alternatives. These center on the manager of projects becoming a leader of people.

Taking Control

Peter Drucker made famous the phrase "Efficiency is doing the right things, but effectiveness is doing the right things in the right way." The right way is often to delegate. Delegation is more than just assigning authority; it is vesting someone with the accountability for clearly defined outcomes.

Incoming telephone calls are a practice constant, but who answers the calls is a variable. If you have established a call back time each day, then 50 to 90 percent of all incoming calls can be handled by the staff. Professors do not come out of class, judges don't come off the bench, baseball players don't come off the field, physicians do not leave their patients, so why should a veterinarian be expected to drop everything because a phone rings? Meetings are another time eater that can follow a published, detailed agenda.

If you cannot delegate, you cannot manage—period. If you are being suckered into making decisions by the upward delegation of your staff, you are wasting time in crisis management. Handling each problem, rather than asking for alternatives from the problem poser, defeats any delegation process. You may be able to do it more quickly and better, but that doesn't train anyone to do it the next time. Delegation works through training, followed by persuading team members that they can do tasks, followed by quiet coaching to refine their techniques so they realize there is latitude in how decisions are made and processes accomplished.

When delegation is the norm, the people on the team must be allowed to say, "I don't know." This is only an indicator that more training is needed, which is a function of leadership. Remember, "We train dogs; we nurture people." The difference between training and nurturing is the persuading and coaching that follow training but precede delegation. The goal is to trust the team so a problem can be referred to a member of the practice staff and the doctor can get back to delivering veterinary medicine.

Delegation

How do you begin to delegate when you are too busy handling everything yourself? You need a system that lets you start to delegate and then keeps the process rolling. Try this daily dozen of delegation:

Prepare yourself

Start keeping a list of your tasks and responsibilities and keep them prioritized. Do the same for each staff member. The total task list should eventually be about 80 percent of the practice's day-to-day routine operational requirements.

Evaluate the staff's capabilities

Each member of the staff was hired for some strength; play to that strength. Rather than "other duties as assigned," end each job description with two phrases: "solve the problem" and "make the improvement." Learn to use the staff's personality traits to help bring out their strengths; know which type of tasks each person *likes* to perform.

Draft a delegation plan

With the preceding two steps in mind, review the principal duties list. Assign or reassign tasks to make delegated work easier but resist the temptation to rely too heavily on the most capable people. Plan supervision, training, and nurturing into the practice plan to make the weaker staff members stronger.

Build in flexibility

Cross-train the staff to prevent illness or quitting from adversely affecting the practice.

Operate efficiently

"Delegating right" means giving the staff enough advanced time to plan, do their other jobs, and still allow the regular system of quality review to be used.

Include some cushions

Build in the time to bypass roadblocks, handle the unexpected, or correct mistakes. Create an annual promotion program for clients and build in a training plan to precede the program. Be flexible enough to know that jobs won't be done exactly the way they have always been done. The end results will be similar, yet better.

Be specific

Take time to communicate concisely and completely. Outcome expectations must be clear; pride comes when expectations are exceeded. Hurried or incomplete instructions cause similar results.

Use delegation as an incentive

Negatively expressed expectations and dwelling on apprehensions are counterproductive. Celebrate attempts to excel, recognize the efforts to meet a challenge, and the dedicated team members will want additional tasks so they can be recognized.

Build team enthusiasm

Celebrate successes, show how they contribute to the whole, and keep momentum growing. Allocate tasks and trust in a fair and equitable manner.

Give rewards

Thank people for efforts as well as progress toward a goal. Praise in public, which means cite each team member's efforts, even for the less glamorous duties.

Support your staff

When members come under pressure by clients, support the staff's actions. Retrain; do not blame. Coping means the leader accepts accountability for whatever happens and accepts the fact that the lack of development of staff proficiency is most often the cause. Be ready to hire additional help when practice success causes growth.

Do regular self-evaluations

Every six months, relist duties and review delegation lists, as in steps one and two. Make the needed modifications to recognize strengths or new emerging specialties.

Payoff

Leadership is delegation. The delegation system will keep running strong if you use it, but it will die if not fed with recognition. Leaders put others before self. They accept that individuals have specific characteristics and needs that must be addressed before they can use these people as resources within the practice. Training to trust means a leader doesn't need to know *how* employees performed tasks but instead must publicly celebrate the outcomes of their efforts each day.

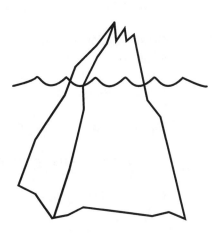

Breaking the Mold

It is a rare veterinary practice that can assume it will be serving exactly
the same client and the same pet market
with the same products and services in six years' time.
—Paraphrased from Jesse Werner

The desk is a dangerous place. When I sit at mine too long, I can't track the veterinary practices I advise, ideas quit flowing, I write less, and I find myself starting to justify habits that prevent me from seeking change. As I visit practices and feel their pressures and frustrations, I begin to form ideas on how to break the mold of old habits. A recent eleven-hour commute from Denver to Mississippi resulted in ideas on the reasons for today's trends, why certain practices sign up for off-site consulting at exceptional costs, and what is really needed for the profession to improve.

The Practice Environment

Fact—The average veterinary practice is never average. The average can be defined as many things, but in the simplest form it is *the best of the worst* or *the worst of the best.* I have never met a veterinarian who strives to make his or her practice either of these.

Fact—Each veterinarian builds an environment based on the sum total of his or her life experiences to date. Most of these experiences include very little structured training on organizational behavior, human resources, or small business operations. Still, there are key characteristics of the practice environment, and these follow a continuum:

Commitment—delegated ⟶ to ⟶ active involvement by ownership

Staff—expensive necessities ⟶ to ⟶ valuable assets and resources

Change—no need to modify ⟶ to ⟶ active listening and action

Operations—process check ⟶ to ⟶ outcome accountability

Involvement—insulated from the staff ⟶ to ⟶ part of the team

Control—highly structured/line ⟶ to ⟶ lateral linkages

Rewards—expected excellence ⟶ to ⟶ timely and specific recognitions

High-performance organizations (HPOs) seldom have a vertical chain of command; the days of the corporate pyramid are over. The HPO allows individuals or small teams to freely act within their areas of accountability and to interact just as freely with lateral groups or individuals (linkages) to improve the workplace. Pride in workmanship is basic to the HPO, and that pride drives an image of quality that every client perceives. In healthcare, we call that pride-based delivery effort CQI (continuous quality improvement).

New Rules for Internal Innovation

The staff members of a practice are valuable jewels that should be cherished; it is up to every veterinarian to polish their facets and show them off to their best advantage. Here are 10 rules for promoting their contribution to practice success:

1. Allow well-defined risks to be taken.
2. Promote flexibility while providing quality care.
3. Waive the standard policies and look to the outcomes.
4. Control the capital by jointly establishing budgets.
5. Create an intrabonded staff team.
6. Leave the staff alone within their accountable areas.
7. Promote the use of volunteers.
8. Give the programs and projects time to mature.
9. Expect some failures; turn them into positive learning experiences.
10. Reward success, celebrate learning, and be responsive.

Project planning is not hard if the boss lets go of the process and lets a staff team explore and develop alternatives. The entire sequence is only six steps (evaluation is required at each step, so the final evaluation is only a summary session):

Identify the problem clearly ⟶
   Team volunteers (3–5 people) ⟶
      Team networks with clients/owners ⟶
         Develops plan (with appropriate budget) ⟶
            Plan (w/staff communication) implemented ⟶
               Recognition of individual & team members ⟶
                  Evaluation for new cycle of problem identification ⟶

Winning Ideas

Traditional marketing creates a need. (Look at McDonald's. Is it a fast food leader or is it just a good forecaster?) Healthcare marketing, on the other hand, creates awareness of a preexisting need. The simple fact is that

Whether you do or whether you don't, you create an image.

Your image is your dignity shadow. Wendy's uses humor to sell food, car dealers use bikinis, and Sears got into trouble by dropping its image of quality to compete in price. NCR has built its electronic data-processing image on innovation, as has Hewlett Packard, but IBM, while less creative than NCR and HP, has kept the lead by projecting an image of service and support. Texaco is even starting to bring back the man with the star to promote its car care service. There has never been a more cost-effective Yellow Pages ad than a 3-inch in-column display with simple phrases like, "evening hours" or "emergencies welcomed anytime." In healthcare, surgicenters and minifamily clinics surfaced in the 1980s because hospitals and physicians did not respond to the clients' demand for responsive emergency care.

When developing the practice image, I've seen everything from soft-sell displays (e.g., a magnifying lens on fleas and worms in front of treatment display) to hard-sell examination room techniques (e.g., cross-sell shampoo). I've seen some practices use couponing while others provide information to educate the client to become a better healthcare consumer. Which technique is better in the long run? Selling spays or shots can get volume, which provides gross for the practice and immediate gratification for clients. This approach has a limited life because it depends on a restricted scope of services and provides a lower net, even though it gives great figures for promotion and practice resale. Uninformed clients look for price first; educated clients look for quality at an affordable value. The service-based practice, the one that is in it for the long run, bases its efforts on client education. The informed consumer will be the one who wants the larger scope of services, will access the facility more often, and will provide a greater net per patient.

The Client Base

Every practice has exactly the client base it deserves. This is simply because it is the client base it has attracted and maintained. Client loyalty in healthcare is often used as a marketing tool, but be aware, only 25 percent of the available clients are a sure bet, and another 25 percent look for the best deal. The middle 50 percent can be influenced by client education. You must know your market.

Clients work from a set of habits, just as practices do. To break the mold that clients have gotten used to takes effort. Primary solicitation in the veterinary marketplace has usually been done with coupons, discounts, or other quick-fix efforts to attract the 25 percent looking for the best deal. Secondary solicitation has been built on public service, by creating an image of dignity in the community that promotes the profession and the awareness of veterinary medical advances. Every catchment area (where the clients come from) has a ceiling. There are just so many people and so many pets living within commuting distance from any given practice. These clients can be gotten by robbery (hard-sell inducements) or creating new awareness (education and information). The short-term results do not always produce long-term effects that profit the practice or profession.

In healthcare, mistrust can kill an effort. Distraction and humor in healthcare marketing are very dangerous; they can tarnish the image of dignity. One veterinarian in every 10 is a huckster; however, even though this affects the image of the reputable practitioners, they cannot fret about this when trying to promote quality healthcare. The smart practice will clearly define objectives before embarking on any client mold-breaking program. Here are some resources for this effort:

Conduct a market survey—Colleges love this opportunity for their students to interview clients.

Problem identification analysis—This can be another college-supported study of community needs.

Client surveys for new or departing clients—Ask the pointed questions that offer answers that could hurt.

Community profiles—Dun & Bradstreet will have a community profile, as well as the Chamber of Commerce, CACI, Equifax, and other demographic firms. These are inexpensive.

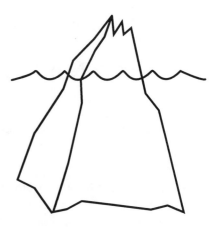

Compare and contrast information—Return on the advertising dollar should be three-fold within a month and four-fold within the quarter; learn to track your efforts.

Beyond Mold-Breaking Rules

The general rules for mold breaking, whether for clients or staff or owners, are based on the elements of quality and trust. They are used in target marketing and change management as well as the daily operations of a veterinary practice:

- James Herriott is still wanted by the consuming pet owner.
- The public must be educated to awareness of needs.
- Relevant information must be provided, not just data.
- Respect is earned, never bought.
- Continuing education is a key to success.
- Consumers must be protected.
- Fraud is fraud; facades are not real.
- Informed clients make informed choices.
- Unjustified statements or statistics are negative factors.
- There are no guarantees, only caring and understanding.
- Disclaimers don't replace quality and caring.
- Continuous quality improvement (CQI) is based on pride being the input of the entire team of providers.

To break the mold, CQI needs to be explored. Authors like Deming, Juran, and Crosby have filled bookstore shelves with books about "total quality management" and "quality is free" concepts. CQI embraces the concept of pride in workmanship, which can be carried into the healthcare field; CQI has been successfully implemented in hospitals for humans. They have found that CQI is not a program but rather a philosophy of operation. It has a dynamic force of its own that enables the staff to become better every day. CQI requires complete and constant leadership support. In the veterinary practice, it empowers every staff member to change the practice for the better, to look for greater efficiency or profit, and to break the mold if it prevents improvement of the healthcare delivery system.

How Not to Cancel Out Cooperation

It isn't hard to manage; it's my way or the highway!
—Famous last words

Good management depends on people doing for people, and in veterinary medicine, it requires practice leadership with a staff-centered focus and a staff with a client-centered focus.

To be successful, a practice manager needs to be a leader, or at least needs to use leadership skills. There are seven major behavior errors made by new hospital managers. If they can be avoided, team cooperation will be enhanced:

Trying to be liked rather than respected

Don't accept favors from other staff members ... don't do special favors in an effort to be liked (do them to help practice productivity) ... don't strive for popular decisions (make them for the good of the client and patient) ... don't be soft about standards and expectations (be clear and consistent) ... don't party or socialize like one of the gang (set the example of professional responsibility) ... have a sense of humor and apply it often!

Failing to ask others for their advice and help

Make other staff members feel a problem is theirs as well as the practice's ... encourage individual thinking and personal commitment to improvement ... never let a person just do a job (make them responsible for solving the problem of the moment) ... make it easy for each person to communicate ideas and accept them as coming from someone who cares about the practice's success ... follow through on staff ideas.

Failing to develop a sense of responsibility in others

Allow each person freedom of expression ... give each person an opportunity to learn some more about the management needs of the practice ... when you give staff responsibility, give them the authority to make unilateral decisions to reach the outcome (let go of control of the process) ... hold each person accountable for jointly predetermined outcome results within the specified time allocated for a project.

Emphasizing the rules rather than the skill

Give a person a job to do and then let him or her do it ... let a staff member own the process and expect that person to make continuous improvements in each task attempted ... train to the knowledge and skills needed for success.

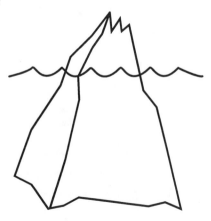

Failing to keep criticism constructive

Accept failure as a training shortfall and an opportunity for change ... instead of making decisions based on hearsay, keep a balanced set of input resources ...

temper and anger are counterproductive (build the dignity of others) ... don't condemn an idea unless you first seek its positive aspects and state them aloud ... don't reiterate past errors and degrade past decision processes (work toward preventing a recurrence of a failure) ... be willing to forgive and make the staff member believe you can also forget.

Not paying attention to staff concerns and complaints

Make it easy for any staff member to come to you ... eliminate chain-of-command concerns ... have a system for grievance and appeal ... help a staff member voice a complaint, and if it involves another person, discuss it with all concerned parties in a quiet room at a quiet time ... practice patience ... always ask the complainer what you can do ... beware of hasty or biased judgments (get the full story firsthand whenever possible) ... let the complainer know what your decision or timetable for a decision is ... double check the results ... stay concerned.

Failure to keep people informed

Let people know where they stand, with you and the practice ... praise people properly (concisely, in public) ... when a project is delegated, let others know who is responsible for the project's success ... keep the staff informed of plans and allow input early in the process, especially before decisions are made ... let people know of changes that may affect them in the future and prevent surprises ... if a change does not affect staff members, tell them anyway so they need not worry.

When you try to manage a team of veterinary healthcare providers, remember: a sense of belonging is as important as a salary. People who believe they belong to a team will cooperate. In fact, considering the salary most practices pay, I would say that belonging and being accountable for patient care is probably more important than salary. If I can leave the veterinary practice manager with one primary principle to embrace and cherish, it would be the following:

A practice manager accepts credit and gives blame,
while a practice leader gives the credit and accepts the blame.

Quality Action Planning

Quality action planning (QAP) is a complex subject that has been covered in many books, but there are a few tenets that may be followed to see the evolution from QAP to healthcare adaptation, as summarized below:

Quality Action Plan
1. Vision (God or architect, you must see it first).
2. Value (teach people how to shop for healthcare).
3. Goals (focus on a few critical issues that really make a difference).
4. Two years to train management, three years for staff.
5. Recognition and reward (go light on the $$).
6. Staff will accept plan *if* they are empowered to change their environment.

Quality Healthcare Planning
1. Clinical outcomes (treat sickness).
2. Service outcomes (client satisfaction).
3. Cost containment (good resource use).
4. Marketing issues (community differentiation).
5. Operational issues (team harmony).
6. Practice pride (restore wellness).

In veterinary medicine, with the community media, new practices, and corporate challengers taking veterinary medicine into the price awareness era of marketing, the question will always arise: "Is cheaper care as good as expensive care?" That decision must be based on three factors:

1. Technical quality = outcome.
2. Service quality = satisfaction.
3. Value = quality + accessibility + service + price.

There are a few veterinary medical traditionalists who wish to take a contract out on those who advertise in the media. While this is not logical to pursue, the local professional meetings are often filled with discussions that could only be resolved by illegal restraint of trade activities. To those who debate this issue, I offer two quotes:

Innovation means the creation of
new values.
—Peter Drucker

First shape the structure, then the
structure will shape us.
—Winston Churchill

Transition to Healthcare

The human healthcare industry of America started to translate total quality management (TQM) principles to its profession in the late 1980s. The first problem it encountered was the word "management"; it did not work. The doctor was the manager of healthcare delivery. So, the term continuous quality improvement (CQI) was born. Some hospitals have even dropped the word "quality" and call their programs continuous improvement (CI); this term suggests every employee is responsible for his or her impact on the system on a daily basis. In hospital research by the American College of Healthcare Executives, repeated studies have shown that CQI requires an uncommon leader, one who is willing to change for the good of the staff and the good of the client and patient. Let's rephrase the 14 principles of W. Edwards Deming, the founder of the TQM concepts, and apply them to veterinary medical practice:

1. Create constancy of purpose (innovation, continuing education, and a single standard of excellence and competency) for the improvement of client service, patient care, and staff harmony.

2. Adopt a practice philosophy of continuous quality improvement; reliable, quality service reduces costs.

3. Cease control of tasks and start building staff pride by giving them control; clients perceive pride as quality.

4. End the practice of evaluating success based on price alone; this mind-set contaminates internal healthcare delivery operations.

5. Putting out fires is not important. Constantly improve the system of staff development and healthcare services.

6. Institute training and retraining by skilled and knowledgeable trainers. It is very difficult to erase improper training.

7. Institute leadership. Discover the barriers that prevent staff members from taking pride in what they do and eliminate the causes.

8. Drive out fear. Preserving the status quo is safe but an economic disaster. Admit mistakes, allow people to take risks, and build on discoveries rather than habits.

9. Break down barriers between staff areas. Good practice leaders cre-

ate an atmosphere of teamwork; they take responsibility for failures rather than dividing the blame.

10. Eliminate slogans, exhortations, and numerical targets for the workforce; if the staff can't reach a goal, they will come to ignore it. Jointly set goals for every quarter in private one-on-one sessions with every staff member.

11. Eliminate the fiscal quotas; they impede quality more than any other single factor. Define quality and train based on the reason for the programs and services, not on the numbers.

12. Remove barriers to pride of workmanship. People are hired because they are motivated and have a good attitude. Build on this trait.

13. Institute a vigorous program of education and retraining; the education must fit people into new jobs and responsibilities.

14. Take action to accomplish the transformation. Use the PDCA cycle: **p**lan, **d**o a 90-day trial, **c**heck benefits to staff/clients/patient/practice, and **a**ccept the new procedure or program.

Regardless of the Deming position, people who access healthcare want quality at a level different from that desired for other goods or services in the community. The definition of quality changes based on the perspective:

Practitioner quality = freedom to act in best interest of patient.
User quality = efficient use of resources consistent with available resources.
Industry quality = meeting requirements while avoiding risks to the institution.
Client quality = exceeding expectations
doing right things right.

Putting It Together

With the above 14 principles in mind, as well as the four healthcare perspectives, we can categorize the critical success factors in the following way:

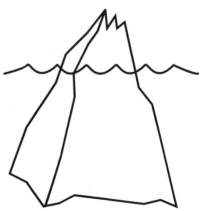

- ◆ reputation for quality
- ◆ unifying vision/focused organization

- financial viability
- market-centered communication plan
- client-centered distribution system
- access to all levels of continuum
- provider support/risk sharing
- system-wide performance standards
- managed care capacity = case management with cost accounting

Now, a reality factor must be injected into this discussion: every veterinary practice believes in quality until the EOM report. To better understand how quality and continuous quality improvement can drive income enhancement activities, look at this simple comparison:

FINANCIAL MANAGEMENT	*Versus*	QUALITY MANAGEMENT
Budget		Quality care plan
Cost control		Quality control
Profit improvement		Quality improvement
Efficiency		Efficacy

The traditional veterinary practice will view CQI as a new program or a project. The reason CQI requires an uncommon leader is that CQI is a process that cannot be ignored in any facet of staff empowerment. It is a new way of looking at issues: tomorrow will be better than today, next week can be improved compared with this week, program enhancements are possible that will make next month better than this month. It is a mind-set assumed by every person in the practice; no one is allowed to be carried. Every person on the team must be willing to take a risk to make an improvement, to leave the status quo, to go where no person has gone before (oops, *Star Trek* is creeping in).

For those who need clarification, there are six phases of a traditional project:

Six Phases of a Traditional Project

1. Enthusiasm
2. Disillusionment
3. Panic
4. Search for the Guilty
5. Punish the Innocent
6. Praise and Honor the Nonparticipants

Though humorous, these phases do exist in some veterinary practices. Risk is avoided at all costs because "if the boss wanted it done she would have told us." Instead, smart practice leaders celebrate the attempt, reward the risk taker, and starve the status quo advocate.

The uncommon leader nurtures creativity and innovation as part of a daily quest toward practice excellence and individual competency. Let's rephrase the six phases into six key parameters:

Six Key Parameters of Continuous Quality Improvement (CQI)

1. Not Available in Powdered Form—it is a total commitment.
2. Not Microwavable—it takes time and effort.
3. No Quick-Fix Shortcut—it requires a step-by-step advancement.
4. Doesn't Fold for Easy Storage—it can't be forgotten, even briefly.
5. No "You May Have Already Won" Messages—change is required.
6. Like Raising Kids, Requires Long-Range Program of Values—yours!

CQI is a systems approach to veterinary practice enhancement. It focuses on both organization and management factors. To best illustrate this concept, look at the following:

Function	Systems Approach	Traditional Practice
Planning	Futuristic	Keep advantage
Management	"What if"	"What now"
Healthcare	Reposition	Expand
Promotion	Client needs	Price competition
Operational review	Quality and value	Job descriptions
Individual review	Performance planning	Appraisals and ratings

Not every practice is ready for the CQI process. It is not a program with a beginning and an end. It is a commitment to change forever. It is a commitment to empower the team to have accountability for outcomes. It is letting go of the control and becoming a motivator, not a taskmaster. Not all practices are ready to grow to this extent; maybe that is why Oregon, Colorado Springs, Toronto, and other locations had a 10 percent practice closure rate in the early 1990s. For those who are ready to grow, they will become the veterinary practice success stories of the next decade.

Personal CQI Checklists

CQI = Continuous Quality Improvement
—Joint Commission for the Accreditation of Healthcare Organizations

Total quality management (TQM) awareness and training programs have proven successful when the leadership releases accountability for outcomes to the employees. In healthcare, this violates the State/Province Practice Act, because doctors can't release cases, so CQI evolved as the alternative. The teams following either approach try to improve organizational processes, which are usually plagued by messy interdepartmental problems. TQM or CQI takes uncommon leadership and a long time to implement, so long that it is often difficult to keep enthusiasm high and coping strategies are needed. A personal CQI checklist often is a great tool to start the process and to keep staff members involved while the leadership gets their goals and objectives into focus.

There are two broad types of job performance enhancers that the personal CQI checklist can help monitor: waste reducers or time savers (such as being on time for activities) and value-added activities (such as calling clients for updates). The first type helps staff members to develop a personal understanding of quality in terms of their immediate work environment. This is valuable in its own right and leads to more effective team participation. But the checklist system is more than a training device. I can bring immediate and substantial improvements in job satisfaction.

A Do-It-Yourself Project

The simplicity of the personal CQI checklist often creates skepticism about its potential benefits. The only way to convince yourself of its usefulness is to try it. You will be surprised by how much and how quickly the checklist can help. You should first notice an improved ability to cope with daily activities and then realize the improvements can be maintained for weeks and months with little or no subsequent effort.

The hardest part is to develop a meaningful checklist. After it is created, actual data collection is almost effortless. You make a check mark when a defect is noticed. It is tempting to develop more elaborate systems that entail more record keeping, but beware. Such elaborate systems add little value and tend to collapse under the data-keeping burden. This seems to be the common thread of failure with many of the prepackaged time management systems. Developing the checklist around what you can personally control or change is critical. It requires insight into job functions and knowledge of the CQI principles.

Look at the incoming tasks first (those that come from others but are yours to resolve). Most can be done quickly but often are delayed due to poor work habits. We have all searched for a medical record, wasting time so that a two-minute entry can be made and the filing completed. We have learned that working harder or faster does not solve the problem of missing medical records. The best route to improvement is to eliminate the wasted effort, obvious and nonobvious, in all its forms.

Composing the personal CQI checklist starts with careful observation and reflection for about two or three weeks. Assemble the categories: borrow some from other checklists if necessary but tailor the words to your own environment. See Figure 5.3 and note that the defects are counted daily to track personal improvement.

If personal CQI checklists are used when the staff are being trained on the principles of CQI, each staff member will gain personal experience and belief in the process. The data could also be used for a simple time series analysis of trends associated with the day of the week or shift staffing. The weekly data charts can be amassed for monthly or long-term monitoring of lateral or vertical relationships.

The simple act of establishing the checklist will cause you to correct some habits immediately (the Hawthorne Effect). Psychological research at the Hawthorne Supply Depot showed if people thought they were being watched or studied, whether they were or not, their performance improved. Some categories will self-correct, and others will need specific attention to resolve. Don't be surprised if the majority of the categories self-correct almost immediately.

The checklist has a calming effect, since by definition everything can't be done at once. The temptation to try is mediated by the check marks the effort causes. Chaos becomes controlled. The checklist permits people to watch themselves as they do things and lets them remove the inefficiencies that are not directly covered in a specific category. There many more categories than are shown in Figure 5.3, such as

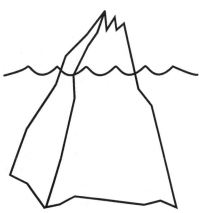

- Failure to meet target dates
- Personal fitness lapses
- Failure to listen closely
- Failure to seek self-improvement weekly
- Making typos, misdialing, or other errors resulting from working too quickly
- Failure to recover promptly from interruptions

Rebecca (the receptionist) Personal CQI Checklist					Week Of: _____				
DEFECT CATEGORY	Mon	Tue	Wed	Thu	Fri	Sat	Sun	TOTAL
Late for Meeting, Appt., or Duty Shift								
Searched for Something Lost or Misplaced								
Delayed Return of Phone Call or Call-back								
Put Small Task on Hold, or Other Procrastination								
Failure to Discard Incoming "Junk" on Front Counter								
Missed a Chance to Clean the Office or Waiting Area								
Unnecessary Inspection of Work								

Definitions:
* **Late** = even by one minute.
* **Search** = more than momentary confusion, includes forgetting a task.
* **Delay** = failure to act at first opportunity.
* **Put on hold** = quick action, like filing a folder, is put off.
* **Discard** = failure to react to clutter, junk is not friendly.
* **Miss a Chance** = any delay in cleaning, dusting, or pickup.
* **Inspection** = checking something already done but attention wasn't paid the first time.

Fig. 5.3. Sample personal CQI checklist.

These concepts are not new. Ben Franklin noted in his autobiography that there are 13 categories to pursue in the search for improved character and behavior: temperance, silence, order, resolution, frugality, industry, sincerity, justice, moderation, cleanliness, tranquility, chastity, and humility. Ben also noted pride often got in the way of improvement of character and behavior, and wrote, "In reality, there is, perhaps, no one of our natural passions so hard to subdue as pride ... even if I could conceive that I had completely overcome it, I should probably be proud of my humility."

Taking a cue from Franklin, here are nine character and behavior traits that should be conquered: unkind humor, defeatism, worry, griping, flustering, sarcasm, unpleasantness, negativity, and dishonesty. You might think a mere checklist could not change behavior or character, but if the checklist is firmly imbedded in your consciousness, the threat of a defect on that list is a strong deterrent to undesirable behavior. Think about it. If you start to feel sorry for yourself, it is defeatism, and the average person will reject the feeling, start another project, or pursue a new goal rather than give him- or herself a check mark.

How Long until Perfection?

How far should anyone go to reduce personal defects? One school of thought says you should never stop. Perfection is the goal; reducing defects annually is the method. But if you believe in CQI, the checklist will change. A change in priorities will cause new items to be added to replace the bad habits that have been corrected. Continual quality improvement will not allow the checklist to be a static set of categories. Some people have a retired category checklist, a list of old habits on a secondary checklist, just in case they revert back to these.

The initial calming effects and the continuous improvement provide the encouragement to continue, but the leadership must support the process. The operational definitions of each category must be defined before the CQI checklist can be used, and that may take some brainstorming with the boss to ensure the categories are realistic. Also, there must be a balance between time waster and value-added activities. Time must be allowed so that new value-added activities can be developed, and a good leader will help maintain the balance. A caring leader will help ensure the goals are *r*ealistic for the environment, *a*ttainable for the person, and *m*easurable (RAM the CQI process).

You Can't Win at Poker Unless You Play the Hand

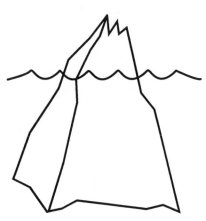

Life consists not in holding good cards but in playing those cards you do hold well.
—*Josh Billings*

The way veterinary services are provided is directly related to the practice's philosophy and the members' feelings of self-worth. It is a lot like playing poker. If you only play when you have a sure win, you lose your ante too often to win for the night. It is not fun to play in this manner.

Choose the Path

Visiting 500-plus veterinary practices, I heard many reasons for why business was slow: "We'd be successful if it weren't for the depressed economy"; "Let me tell you, I'd be making it if it weren't for the interest rates I'm paying"; "I'd be on top of the world today if I could just find the right associate"; "You know, I'd really be successful if it weren't for all those new graduates flooding the market"; "We would expand if it weren't for those zoning codes." This abridged list of excuses is made by externalists. Externalists blame some condition or other people for their failures. This refusal to accept responsibility places success outside their grasp.

On the other hand internalists are performance oriented. They accept accountability for their successes, failures, and actions. They do not cry over spilt milk; they just look for another cow to milk. They take the hand life deals and play it to the very best of their ability. They are the ones who are not afraid to say, "I don't know," or as Harry Truman's Oval Office sign read, "The buck stops here."

Essentially, there are only two paths of action in veterinary practice management, or life for that matter: performing and making excuses. Practice managers must decide which path they will lead their practice teams down. We can predict the amount of failure any individual or team will experience by a simple formula:

People fail in direct proportion to their willingness to accede to
socially acceptable excuses for failure.

The problem with most veterinary practice management assessments is the traditional dictum "well, my practice is different" or "your clients are different," or "my staff are different." It ain't so, folks! Any one of these excuses encourages failure if repeated to the staff every day.

Philosophy of Success

The philosophy of success lies in the philosophy of management, and we need to define management in terms that allow success to be achieved. For the purpose of veterinary practice, let me share a definition that works for me:

Management is the art of attaining measurable goals and objectives
with and through the voluntary cooperation, enthusiasm,
and effort of other people.

Mike Vance, of Disney fame, said, "Mothering is managing." It is not the art of winning that is a cornerstone in management but rather clearly communicating and diligently monitoring tasks and goals, then fairly rewarding the people who achieve them because they have made a commitment based on personal interest and the good of the organization.

Management is not mothering, but mothering is management. No mother waits six months to give her kid a performance appraisal for trying to dry the cat in the clothes dryer. Every day mothers manage conflict, correct and guide behavior, motivate peer social groups, set goals for others, and get the dishes washed, diapers changed, and garbage taken out (and still manage to be loved).

The KSA Approach

One of the foremost leadership and management courses available today rates all performance based on only three factors: knowledge, skills, and attitude. This is the KSA approach, and the elements are critical.

Knowledge is the foundation upon which we build. It allows alternatives to be seen and explored. Enough knowledge can help overcome the bias and bigotry of the school of hard knocks.

Skills are simply the ability to share knowledge. They represent the transformation of mental warehousing into action that achieves personal goals and objectives in a timely and effective manner.

Attitude is the cornerstone upon which leadership and management rely to make knowledge and skills useful to the organization. Attitude helps the team select the right path to success.

These aid leadership when shared, improve management when used personally, and are rewarding when used routinely. We can apply the KSA concept of management excellence to the analogy of the poker hand. Knowledge of the deck and game rules does not provide the skill to play the game. That skill comes from repetition, mistakes, and disasters. The need to discover success carries with it the need to experience failures. A skillful player accumulates knowledge with each failure, in cards or in life. But the real secret to a suc-

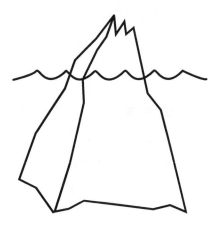

cessful poker game is the attitude of the player. A good player bluffs occasionally, but that is only one of many skills brought to the table. The tenacity to keep trying, the knowledge that the cards cannot be blamed, and the skill of reading the body language of others result from the player's attitude of self-accountability and personal responsibility for all actions.

Attitude Adjustment Exercise

Most every problem encompasses an opportunity, and most every solution can be negative or positive. In the left column of the following exercise are negative situations, and on the right are the opportunities to excel. Your task is to fill in the blanks (team brainstorming is allowed).

SOLVE THESE CHALLENGES
(*team brainstorming is allowed*)

SITUATION

OPPORTUNITY

Your house has been robbed, all the valuables are gone.

Call a friend and plan that dream vacation with the excess insurance money from the unneeded "stuff" that was stolen.

Mrs. Jones calls the practice and states that the treatment is not working at all.

_____
_____
_____

You discover the first leash chain dent on the new front door.

Throw a party because you don't have to worry about the first dent anymore.

The new animal caretaker is going to quit unless you can make the work more rewarding.

_____
_____
_____

Your stock dividend is delayed.

Tell a friend that your broker is saving vacation money for you.

Accounts receivable are $23,000 for the last fiscal year.

_____
_____
_____

In veterinary practice, our formal education gave us the knowledge we need, and the hours we've spent at the exam or surgery table have given us the skills. Attitude is what separates the successful practice from the average practice. In the last situation above, the accounts receivable may be less than 1 percent, which is a reason to celebrate in most practices. It means there is excellent client bonding by the staff and practice. What was your first response this example?

Moving Mountains

To many veterinary healthcare professionals, management is like trying to move mountains ... it is done in very small increments, making the goal seem impossible to reach. But it does not have to be a traumatic experience if we remember a few basic principles. The attitudes of the veterinarians and the hospital manager set the tone for the implementation of the practice philosophy as well as the team's approach to facing adversity. There must be no blame—problems must be opportunities for new goals and objectives. It is this attitude that keeps us in the game, that lets us see where we can make changes and lead our teams to success.

Smart leaders provide alternatives to their teams that they personally embrace, but they do not tell the teams which one they prefer. The good leader fully embraces the team's best shot at an acceptable alternative and helps the team develop an implementation plan that requires individual commitment rather than "taskings." Remember:

When it is everyone's responsibility, no one is accountable.

Accountability relates to the outcome expectation, not the process. Old-time managers (and traditional consultants) are heavy into job descriptions, procedure manuals, and standards for process. These are important for training new people to a level of healthcare competency, but they are are *only* the starting point in the New American Veterinary Practice.

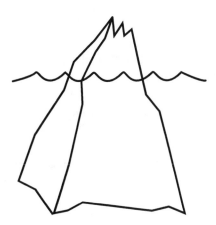

Understanding Excuses

A member of your staff says he can't complete a task because someone else on the staff hasn't done the job he asked him to do. A client keeps putting off the surgery date for Fifi, ostensibly because she is too committed to other community activities. The practice owner says she can't give you an answer until she talks to the bookkeeper; in the meantime, the project, which will help the practice, is stalled. Excuses are usually only reasons to stall progress. Excuses tend to build the management mountains higher, and they never make the trail any easier.

Excuses may be legitimate, or they may be used to shield the truth. When an excuse interferes with progress—yours or the practice's—it is smart not to accept it at face value. But as a practice leader, you must assume there is some truth in any excuse. You will only put the other person on the defensive if you project an "I don't believe you" attitude. If the excuse maker works for you, take a problem-solving approach. For example, suggest that the two of you talk to the person is preventing a job from being done. You'll be able to gauge the truthfulness of your employee's excuse by his or her reaction.

If the other employee is not to blame, the excuse maker will probably communicate discomfort by avoiding eye contact, hesitating before answering, or making yet another excuse such as "I don't think Mary is free right now, but I'll check with her as soon as she is." If you are dealing with a valued and usually reliable employee, simply reiterate the importance of the task and the need to get it completed as soon as possible. Make it clear that the mountain is in the path of practice progress and the team will need to climb it. He or she will probably get the message.

Sometimes excuses are used to register dissatisfaction. An employee whose excuses have become more frequent may be hesitant to communicate the real problem. You will have to convey that it is safe for the employee to be honest. You might say, for example, "I value you and I would like to know if something is bothering you and preventing you from doing your usual good work." To give this person an opportunity to say what is on his or her mind may well bring an issue you were unaware of out into the open. If you are willing to address the issue fairly, chances are the excuses will stop.

Accountability must be assumed by the team. As stated in Vol. 2 of this series, the best method for emphasizing this is to add two lines to every job description *after* the introductory hire period (after the employee has learned the initial job description and expectations of excellence and is competent in the routine procedures):

1. Meet the challenge—solve the problem!
2. See the need—make the improvement!

Dealing with Client Excuses

When clients build mountains from molehills, you can use the approach outlined in the preceding section. Assume the excuse has some element of truthfulness, ask the client a question, analyze the response, and then react in a logical fashion, but substitute persuasiveness for directness.

If, for example, the client uses the "I'm too busy" excuse as a reason for not accessing needed healthcare for a pet, sympathize with the predicament that the client is experiencing. Then turn the excuse around to find out if there is a bigger obstacle. There may be a great fear of the anesthetic risk to the pet or the worry about a large surgical expense. You might suggest a before- or after-hours drop-off that better fits the client's schedule, or a time payment system to meet his or her budget.

If your remark catches the client by surprise and there is no immediate response, you can invite frankness. For example, "I sense there is another concern that is preventing us from doing the surgery that Fifi needs. If I or my staff have done something to make you worry about the procedure, I would really like to know so that I can do something about it." If no problem exists, the client will probably be more willing to share other personal concerns to alleviate your self-blame. Even better, the client may set up a time to drop off Fifi and "ask a few more questions."

"I can't afford it" does not always mean an insurmountable mountain has appeared on the horizon. It may mean the checkbook is at home, the charge card is full, or payday isn't until next week. If you question what clients really mean, the answers may indicate problems that can be resolved. Regardless, the concern you show clients will improve their bond to the practice.

Excuses from the Boss

Being direct or persuasive is more difficult when the person making the excuse has power over you. Still, if what you ask is important to you or to the productive functioning of the practice, it is worthwhile to get some direct answers. If you are waiting for funding for a project, for example, suggest that the two of you discuss what can be done to spend the money wisely or to implement the project most efficiently once the funds become available. If your boss is unwilling to help, you may

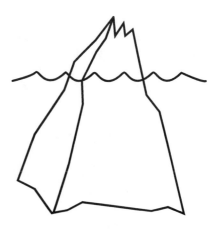

have to ask directly whether or not the project has his or her ongoing support.

The other method for dealing with a boss who makes excuses instead of decisions can be used only if you are secure in your position in the practice. If you are invaluable, remember the adage "it is always easier to ask for forgiveness rather than for permission." If an idea will benefit the practice, you might be able to make the decision, implement the idea, see it working, and evaluate the improvements before the boss notices. Then you can enjoy the fame and fortune as you ask for forgiveness.

The Finger Pointer's Excuse

If a person frequently makes excuses, he or she may simply be a con artist. Someone who routinely builds mountains in the practice's path should not be pampered. Be prepared to fire the employee, refer the client to another practice, or leave the practice if the finger pointer is the boss. Why? Because people who are that manipulative are only prepared to help you if their self-interest matches yours. That can be frustrating and unproductive.

Management Is Control of a Resource

As in any mountain assent, there are tools and training available to make the climb safer and more rewarding. The most important tool in a veterinary practice is the strength of the healthcare delivery team. Every member is a resource with an opinion. If we take the time to recognize that the staff care about the success of the practice, then we can use their input to conquer adversity.

1. Never ignore an idea because it has a flaw. If a perfect solution can't be found, then a compromise must be considered in light of the benefits. As we reevaluate the idea, the original flaw may just disappear from the equation.

2. Never reject an alternative because you won't get the credit you deserve for thinking of it. This could also be called the *Miracle on 34th Street* syndrome. The recognition is not as important as the long-term benefit of improving the team or the patient's welfare.

3. Never discard an idea because it is impossible. Ignoring the impossible enabled us to fly, use electrocautery, and take X rays.

4. Never reject an alternative because your mind is already made up or

because it doesn't fit into your way of doing things. Biases, which are formed by past experiences, may restrict the practice's future. It is amazing how we lock out alternatives just because there was not an opportunity to utilize them in a previous situation.

5. Never disregard an idea because it's illegal. Waivers are granted every day by the zoning commission, and laws are changed by the courts and legislatures on a routine basis. Why is it that we believe the rules of a previous generation are inviolate even though we see exceptions occurring daily?

6. Never refuse to consider an alternative just because you don't have the money, workforce, muscle, or months to achieve it. These are all factors that can be overcome if we set goals and objectives with measurable milestones to gauge our progress.

7. Never discard an alternative just because it will create conflict. The real challenge of change is that it usually meets with resistance, whether the change be shorter daytime hours so we can open at night, increasing the fee schedule, or just papering the wall with a brighter pattern vinyl. The immediate conflict must be weighed against the long-term objectives of the practice.

8. Never reject an idea just because it might fail. In the human health-care industry, it is estimated that less than 20 percent of all marketing ideas are ever implemented, and only half of those become successes. The 10 percent that do succeed make the hospital into the community leader, a place where we want our facilities. To fail only means we tried, but lack of failure usually means we have quit growing and learning, which means we have died, even if we don't realize it yet.

Moving Mountains Cycle

The following figure illustrates how, when faced with a challenge, you can move mountains. The term "public commitment" means letting your practice team know what you want and where you hope to go. Share your wishes and dreams, and let the team buy into them. Those who do not dare to dream doom themselves to a very boring existence of mediocrity.

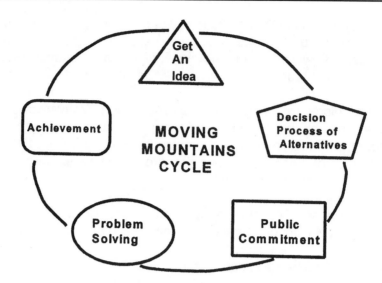

Moving mountains can be fun, almost as fun as watching the expressions on our colleagues faces when we achieve the improbable. And when we achieve the impossible, watching the expressions of our staff when the rewards are shared. Let your staff help you move those mountains and have fun doing it.

Building Your Practice Team Flag

We rally around symbolism. We believe in the effectiveness of a logo to establish a community identity. Americans salute the Stars and Stripes. In the Lone Star state, people fly the state flag with pride. What is the flag that flies in your veterinary practice? What elicits pride?

The client-centered habits on which most practices are built soon shift to a bottom line fixation on the profit and loss statements. Then the flag of caring for clients changes to one of caring about the average transaction fee. The staff start to fret about their bonuses rather than client satisfaction. The veterinary practice of today must do more with less. The margin of profit has dwindled. A business cannot spend the gross; it can only spend the net. The reason for the dwindling net varies from increased community competition, to veterinary price wars, to poor management techniques. Regardless of the cause, the best tools available to change trends are the human resources within the practice. Veterinarians work hard to produce the gross, but the paraprofessionals are the ones who increase the practice net.

Build a New Practice Flag for Tomorrow

Every practice owner can change the practice flag. It is more than a slogan like "Sharing the caring" or "We care for a pet as if it were our own." It should be based on a systematic approach to quality healthcare, continuity of care, and use of veterinary extenders. Veterinary extenders are simply those people or things that give the veterinarian more time for patient care, whether they be forms, policies, or veterinary technicians who provide quality patient and client care. Let's look at the elements that need to be included in a quality practice F-L-A-G:

Followers   Every team requires players, else you cannot call it a team—they must be willing to play by the rules established for the game.

Leadership   Every team needs someone to make the hard decisions, set the pace, and provide the feedback on activities.

Attitude   The attitude of concern for excellence must be seen at all levels, from the followers to the leaders.

Goals   Any team needs to know where it is going, where it can be recognized for making a successful score.

Followers

Believe it or not, psychologists tell us that 50 percent of the American workforce have the personality that prefers predictable, steady, routine work. Another 16.3 percent of the American workforce prefers lifestyles that are very structured and a workplace loaded with policy statements and procedure manuals. This means the veterinary practice manager has a two in three chance of hiring a process-oriented follower. By definition, this type of follower must have a leader to be effective and comfortable within a work environment.

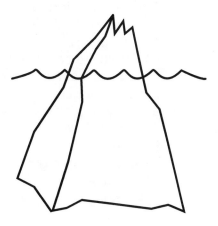

Followers need to have a flag to rally behind. They need to know what the expectations are, where the practice is going, and what determines competence. The basic issue in healthcare delivery is competency. The range is not excellent, outstanding, good, fair, weak, or poor.

Every text on healthcare delivery states a single standard of performance is necessary, and within the American Animal Hospital Association consulting program, that is called competency. If staff members are below competency, they need training. If they are incompetent, they need to be fired! Above competency, which must equated with excellence (considering the forensic nature of healthcare delivery), is a category I call "ready to train others." This category recognizes the training ability of the best followers to help improve their team members' performance.

Leadership

Members of a veterinary practice staff want to believe they are in a caring profession; they want to be recognized as representing the best in healthcare delivery. When staff members know they share the practice philosophy, that they are practicing it, they know they are rallying behind the flag of the practice owner or veterinarian. The flag represents the core values of the practice. When decisions are made by employees using these core values, only accolades should be given. No one should ever feel the standards are inconsistent. These are the flag characteristics of a quality practice and are the keys to effective practice leadership and team building.

The staff must be able to depend on the veterinarian for support of the practice's standards, even if they upset a client. If the doctor learns to say, "I'm sorry, it was my fault, we initiated that program to help the majority of our clients; I'm sorry we hadn't planned for your situation ...," then the staff will feel supported by the leader. As the boss treats the staff, so will the staff treat the clients. The leader's vision and dream will be supported when the team is led by example.

Attitude

The simple rule in leading a team is "Whether you think you can, or whether you think you can't, you make it come true." A leader with a positive attitude builds on the strengths for which each individual was hired. We don't hire people for their weaknesses. A leader with a positive attitude trusts team members to solve problems instead of waiting for other people to act. Leaders with a positive attitude focus on patient advocacy, a quality of care issue, and speak up for the needs of the pet. They let clients get involved in decisions about the level of care for needed for their pets.

Leaders with a great attitude remember that the only team members who stumble and make mistakes are those who are moving forward and trying something new. This is a characteristic of learning. Those who never make mistakes and never stumble are standing still and playing it safe. This will not lead to growth.

Goals

Everyone wants practice growth, but there are many who do not realize that direction is needed for orderly team advancement. While many practices say they have not had time to define clear, concise, and embraceable objectives, they have found the time to train new staff members on a recurring basis. High staff turnover is often symptomatic of staff who do not identify with the practice standards.

Every team must have a goal. All team sports have expectations that are clearly defined, from what the team wears to the size of the playing field to how team members are to treat others while they try to score. The team captain and the coach tell team members what is expected and how they are to work together to make the score. Some teams need more direction than others. A practice team must be in it for the long haul, not just a four-hour game. A good leader keeps the goals and objectives clearly defined and in front of the team. The purpose of the goal is also explained to increase motivation. A great leader also puts him- or herself into the team members' shoes and tries to see the challenges from their perspective.

Rally around the Flag

George M. Cohan brought a flutter to the heart as he sang "You're a Grand Old Flag." You can do this for your practice. To get your staff to support the practice, you must appeal to their emotions, which requires your sharing personal beliefs and making a personal commitment to the staff and their goals. It requires stretching beyond your personal comfort zone and taking off your shoes before you try walking in theirs. To make success happen,

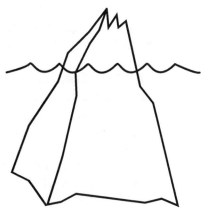

- You must understand that the needs of staff members (not their wants) must be met before they will be dedicated to meeting the demands you have for the practice.
- You must find out what excites each person, what each person wants to achieve, and how each person wants to contribute to the practice.

■ You need to tailor your staff utilization plan to the strengths of the team members.

■ You must be willing to build on small easy successes before you attempt to take on those big challenges.

■ You must be willing to commit resources to build the staff's self-image before they will buy into saluting the practice standards, or flag.

Setting the Vision

There are many reasons to build a team flag and to pursue continuous quality improvement (CQI), but the bottom line is that it rewards our staff. It is used to increase net, and the net can be shared with the team, but the members' pride in their performance is the real reward. With the low wages veterinarians usually pay, and the dedication of the staff who join the team, the ability to recognize the staff's efforts makes the difference between turnover and tenure. Look to your practice image and see if it is something others can rally around.

Both clients and staff want to believe in the quality of a practice's care. Promote continuous quality improvement and the staff will be proud to represent the practice. When the staff are proud, the clients become proud. When the clients become proud, your practice will develop a market niche in your community.

Inside the Veterinary Practice

We have seen the innovative and creative people in veterinary practices: the technician who is also a dog obedience trainer and, through the practice, offers free classes in the practice parking lot; the receptionist who develops a color coding system for patient records that allows easy reference for follow-up or reminders; or the veterinarian who offers assistance to local healthcare institutions for the development of animal-facilitated therapy programs and greatly increases the sphere of practice influence and goodwill among more economically stable populations. The climate for innovation and creativity requires

■ The leadership to have a clear and consistent vision.

■ The practice to have concise quarterly and long-term goals and objectives.

■ Individual accountability and responsibility, instead of blame and red tape.

■ Freedom to make mistakes during the testing and operating phases.

■ A reward system that is tied to the contributions to the practice.

One of the key elements for developing such an environment within your practice is the integrated annual plan. Not a series of gimmicks from seminars or journals, but an actual annual plan, based on the annual business cycle and the three-year business plan. The projected outcomes must be clearly identified, the programs must have substance, and any new ideas must be fit into the flow; monthly and recurring in-service education enhances the skills and knowledge of each individual. Each member of the staff who knows what is expected by the end of the year can have accountability for accelerating the process whenever it touches his or her sphere of influence.

The innovative practice staff must march to a different drummer. In school and traditional businesses, time and task are considered constants, which makes achievement the variable. To the innovators, the dream is the constant; they'll do anything to make their projects work. They'll work underground and after-hours. They know it's easier to ask for forgiveness than for permission, and they'll build a network of people to help them. The successful innovators, while coming to work each day, are willing to be fired rather than lose their dreams, yet they will be realistic about the ways to achieve them. They learn never to bet on a race unless they are running in it. These are *work enthusiasts,* not workaholics who act out of fear.

Successful innovators are never surprised to win, never expect to fail, yet are not afraid to fail. They need to have a positive self-image but know that self-image has nothing to do with potential. It has everything to do with performance. A positive self-image allows the innovators to question the events that occur around them and allows them to believe they can improve them, for their boss or the organization. James M. Utterback, in *Technological Innovation for a Dynamic Economy,* pointed out that initial uses of innovations tend to be small, and often expensive. For example, ice was first manufactured at great expense and danger for the inland South, where harvested ice was prohibitively expensive, and rayon, although difficult to dye, was first produced and used for a uniform filament for incandescent lights and only later was used as a high-performance tire cord.

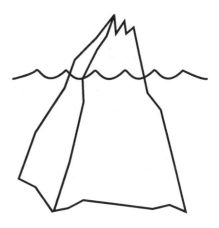

The reward system can be tangible, like a percentage of increased income being placed into a fund for new business development within the practice, or intangible, like formal acknowledgment and posted pictures of the employee. Whatever the system, the reward must provide time or capital to the innovators to allow their creativity and innovation to flourish. Regardless of the reward, staff members' inspiration and innovation may result in mistakes on occasion, and the method of dealing with these errors can promote or stifle innovation and creativity. A wise man once said, "Make a hundred first mistakes each day, and you'll learn quickly, which is good; start making mistakes for a second time and that is bad." This represents the difference between management and leadership, and between planners and reactors. Good leaders are also good planners with a vision for where the team and practice should go.

Build It and They Will Come

So how do you build an innovative team? First, the planners are the doers. There is no manager telling staff what to do. Everyone pitches in to get a job done. The team has a sense of ownership. It owns the problems and joys of creating success. The team members are recruited by the planners (leaders), not assigned by a supervisor. All team members are considered members of a learning organization (remember, knowledge doubles every two years in veterinary medicine; old knowledge is often obsolete). They take the personal risk to turn a vision into a reality for the good of the practice. The team needs to be allowed to distribute rewards based on the involvement of and risk taken by the people who made the outcome a success.

Often, many practices find it easier to describe their products or services than to identify the important customers and their needs. The easiest marketing plan is one for a market made up of only a few clients. We don't have that luxury in a veterinary practice. The market is a variety of often stressed clients who need to have their needs met: dual-income couples, single parents, breeders, retirees, newly marrieds, first-pet owners, owners of aged family member animals, people without discretionary income, and even a few with more money than the national debt! Flexibility is required of staff members on a day-by-day and moment-by-moment basis. Just "doing the job" is seldom adequate. A leader develops the environment where doing the job is taught during the 90-day probationary period immediately after hiring and then problem solving is the expectation thereafter. The progressive practitioner will spend quality time brainstorming ideas with the practice staff or thinking out loud with team members about needs, wants, and innovations. Doing this in an environment conducive to innovation and creativity will yield results and cash flow that will take the practice successfully into the next millennium and beyond.

Build the learning organization, and they will come.
Promote the learning, and innovation will follow.
Innovation and creativity are a market edge.
A market niche yields net income.
Net income causes smiles.
Just do it.
Now!

Application Exercise

As stated in the Introduction, mind mapping is an excellent technique not only for generating ideas but also for developing intuitive capabilities. Use the iceberg ideas you have added on the odd-numbered pages and the concepts you have drawn from this chapter to expand the following mind map.

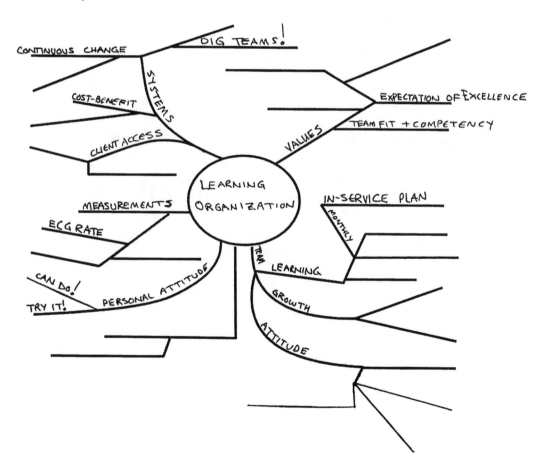

Issues

- Does your practice hold regular staff meetings?
- Does the management talk at the staff for the entire meeting?
- Did you try the Volume 1 meeting management system (see Vol. 1, Appendix A, pp. 141–44) but it fell into disuse?

Action

- Change the system!
- Power to the people!

In many veterinary practices, meeting agendas become routine, and the meeting ceases to be productive. This is often because when the staff meetings were started the practice was too small to have effective meetings. This appendix is an alternative to gripe sessions. It puts the rubber on the road. It has been most successful in larger practices, but a few small practices have adapted it and found the basic concepts very useful.

The *Do It Group* (DIG) means put up or shut up in management terms, but in leadership terms, it means "we trust you to initiate projects for the good of the practice, for the benefit of the client, and for patient advocacy." The signal to start is when three people agree on some issue—any issue—and leaders control the process by ensuring the outcome success measurements are understood before the DIG starts.

This is an exciting concept and has worked very well in human healthcare. There are some hospitals that have papered the walls of their staff cafeterias with DIG activities and success stories ... isn't this a goal to strive for in your practice?

DIG BOARD

DIG = Do It Group

Project/Task/Idea	Sign-up for Three Volunteers BEFORE starting			DIG Start Date	Finish Date	Cat
	1	2	3			

Concepts

- *Anyone* can put something (an idea, task, project, etc.) in the left column.
- When three staff members have put their names by a project, the clock starts ticking, but only after three have entered their names (record the start date when the third person signs the board).
- When the project is finished, or at the end of 60 days, whichever is first, the completion date is recorded and rated (categories: 1 = done and happy, 2 = done but we spun off some other DIG projects, and 3 = we did not finish, and we spun off smaller DIG projects).

Why the DIG Board? Let Us Show You!

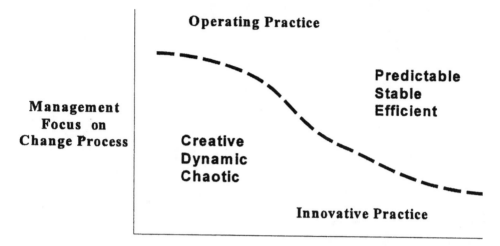

Time - Rate of Change

Early Phase	Middle Phase	Later Phases
Ideas	Efficiency	Rigid Process
Entrepreneurial	Alignments	Bureaucracy
Highly Creative	Turf Wars	High Efficiency
Reward "new"	Reward "same"	Reward "safe"

Innovation and Creativity

- The DIG Board allows the early phase to continue.
- The management focus is on people—doing well comes with time.
- The fear is not of failure but of stasis. DIG Boards encourage dynamic thinking.
- Celebration of the attempt of the DIG reinforces creativity.
- Change is chaos—get used to it. Begin today!

Training Profile

As you read the statements in this profile, select the response that best fits the way you conduct, or plan to conduct, the in-service training in your practice. Some of the statements focus on your ideas about how training ought to be done. If you have not yet developed and taught an in-service session, try to respond to each statement based on the philosophy of your practice.

When you determine your response, just note the number on the line to the left of each statement. Do not look at part two until you have completed this section.

Note: This profile is intended for the trainer only. It shouldn't be graded by others; it is a self-help guide.

___ 1. I follow the in-service training plan exactly to keep the subject matter on schedule and to make sure that all parts of the program are covered.
   (3—Very much like me; 2—Much like me; 1—Somewhat like me; 0—Hardly like me)

___ 2. I give the participants a copy of the in-service training outline so that they will know what is happening and when.
   (3—Very much like me; 2—Much like me; 1—Somewhat like me; 0—Hardly like me)

___ 3. When a staff member disagrees strongly with something I say when training, I check with others to find out if the disagreement is shared.
   (3—Very much like me; 2—Much like me; 1—Somewhat like me; 0—Hardly like me)

___ 4. I think staff members should be tested on the facts covered during any in-service training event.
   (3—Strongly agree; 2—Agree; 1—Disagree; 0—Strongly disagree)

___ 5. If a staff member fell asleep during a sit-down training session, I would likely ignore him/her since there is probably a good reason for being so tired.
   (3—Very much like me; 2—Much like me; 1—Somewhat like me; 0—Hardly like me)

___ 6. Staff members should be able to see how the material being taught will help them with their daily duties as well as how it will help the practice.
   (3—Strongly agree; 2—Agree; 1—Disagree; 0—Strongly disagree)

___ 7. Staff in-service participants should receive grades from the trainer.
   (3—Strongly agree; 2—Agree; 1—Disagree; 0—Strongly disagree)

___ 8. I use group participation methods like role-playing and discussion groups when I conduct in-service training in order to get the staff totally involved.
   (3—Very much like me; 2—Much like me; 1—Somewhat like me; 0—Hardly like me)

___ 9. Some staff members have to be motivated by negative methods.
   (3—Strongly agree; 2—Agree; 1—Disagree; 0—Strongly disagree)

___10. Trainers cannot do a good job unless they are experts in what they are training.
> (3—Strongly agree; 2—Agree; 1—Disagree; 0—Strongly disagree)

___11. The entire staff should be given reports on how a staff member does in a subject.
> (3—Strongly agree; 2—Agree; 1—Disagree; 0—Strongly disagree)

___12. I go into depth in those parts of the in-service subject(s) where staff interest is high, even if other parts of the in-service will have less time.
> (3—Very much like me; 2—Much like me; 1—Somewhat like me; 0—Hardly like me)

___13. I find the best teaching methods for me are discussions with open-ended questions that have no "wrong" answers.
> (3—Very much like me; 2—Much like me; 1—Somewhat like me; 0—Hardly like me)

___14. When a staff member disagrees with an idea from the in-service, I repeat the concept so that he/she will agree with it.
> (3—Very much like me; 2—Much like me; 1—Somewhat like me; 0—Hardly like me)

___15. One of the primary benefits of in-service training is to inspire staff toward the practice goals.
> (3—Strongly agree; 2—Agree; 1—Disagree; 0—Strongly disagree)

___16. If the trainer is interesting, tests should not be necessary.
> (3—Strongly agree; 2—Agree; 1—Disagree; 0—Strongly disagree)

___17. I spend a great deal of time beginning each in-service getting to know who wants to work with whom during the training.
> (3—Very much like me; 2—Much like me; 1—Somewhat like me; 0—Hardly like me)

___18. If a staff member falls asleep during the sit-down training, I feel I should reprimand him/her to set an example for the others.
> (3—Very much like me; 2—Much like me; 1—Somewhat like me; 0—Hardly like me)

___19. If someone strongly disagrees with something I said, I should deal directly with this challenge to my authority so the course will not get out of hand.
> (3—Strongly agree; 2—Agree; 1—Disagree; 0—Strongly disagree)

___20. In my sessions, I feel strongly that a personal, one-on-one interaction between me and a participant is extremely important.
> (3—Very much like me; 2—Much like me; 1—Somewhat like me; 0—Hardly like me)

___21. When a staff member strongly disagrees with something I said, I ask for his/her point of view so that others can decide for themselves which ideas are correct.
> (3—Very much like me; 2—Much like me; 1—Somewhat like me; 0—Hardly like me)

___22. The practice owner should not be told how staff members are doing in the coursework.
> (3—Strongly agree; 2—Agree; 1—Disagree; 0—Strongly disagree)

__23. When a staff member strongly disagrees with something I have said, I restate the point as a question, perhaps using different words or examples, so that he/she will better understand the point.
(3—Very much like me; 2—Much like me; 1—Somewhat like me; 0—Hardly like me)

__24. I should follow the in-service outline exactly as written since it is hospital policy once it is written and approved.
(3—Strongly agree; 2—Agree; 1—Disagree; 0—Strongly disagree)

__25. I do my best training when I am working from a loose outline—going with the flow of the staff's questions and discussions.
(3—Very much like me; 2—Much like me; 1—Somewhat like me; 0—Hardly like me)

__26. It is often necessary to criticize one participant quite strongly in order to get an important point across to the rest of a resistant staff.
(3—Strongly agree; 2—Agree; 1—Disagree; 0—Strongly disagree)

__27. The main purpose of in-service training is to get subject matter across to the participants so they know it well.
(3—Strongly agree; 2—Agree; 1—Disagree; 0—Strongly disagree)

__28. I prefer self-evaluation exercises in which only the staff member sees the results.
(3—Very much like me; 2—Much like me; 1—Somewhat like me; 0—Hardly like me)

__29. When a staff member is doing something different from what the rest of the participants are working on (e.g., reading vendor inserts), I feel it is necessary to get that staff member to join the course activity.
(3—Very much like me; 2—Much like me; 1—Somewhat like me; 0—Hardly like me)

__30. In general, when training in a multipractice consolidation, it is unnecessary for the participants to introduce themselves to each other at the beginning of the course.
(3—Strongly agree; 2—Agree; 1—Disagree; 0—Strongly disagree)

__31. Getting subject matter across is more important than whether or not the participants enjoy the session.
(3—Strongly agree; 2—Agree; 1—Disagree; 0—Strongly disagree)

__32. A trainer must believe in the importance of the subject matter he/she is teaching. If the participants in the in-service do not share in that belief, it is the trainer's job to convince them of its value.
(3—Strongly agree; 2—Agree; 1—Disagree; 0—Strongly disagree)

__33. I find that tests are a necessary motivational device. Staff members learn more when they know they will be tested.
(3—Very much like me; 2—Much like me; 1—Somewhat like me; 0—Hardly like me)

__34. In general, participants in an in-service are not capable of accurately evaluating the job done by the trainer.
(3—Strongly agree; 2—Agree; 1—Disagree; 0—Strongly disagree)

__35. All in all, lecture is still the best method of covering the subject properly.

(3—Strongly agree; 2—Agree; 1—Disagree; 0—Strongly disagree)

___36. When a participant is engaged in an activity different from what the rest of the group is doing (e.g., reading instead of listening), I overlook it and work with the other staff members.

      (3—Very much like me; 2—Much like me; 1—Somewhat like me; 0—Hardly like me)

___37. In my sessions, I work with each individual in a different way in order to meet each one's unique needs

      (3—Very much like me; 2—Much like me; 1—Somewhat like me; 0—Hardly like me)

___38. The most important factor in deciding which teaching method I will use for a specific topic is what I feel comfortable with.

      (3—Strongly agree; 2—Agree; 1—Disagree; 0—Strongly disagree)

___39. I believe the primary purpose of in-service training is to get staff members ready to meet the needs of clients and doctors.

      (3—Very much like me; 2—Much like me; 1—Somewhat like me; 0—Hardly like me)

___40. When a staff member strongly disagrees with something I said, I listen carefully to try to find something he/she is saying that I can agree with.

      (3—Very much like me; 2—Much like me; 1—Somewhat like me; 0—Hardly like me)

___41. I try to make sure that the staff participants enjoy the course I am conducting.

      (3—Very much like me; 2—Much like me; 1—Somewhat like me; 0—Hardly like me)

Do not proceed until all 41 questions have been answered.
Please proceed if all 41 questions have been answered.

Scoring Instructions

1. Transfer your answers from the questionnaire to the appropriate spaces below:

	A		B
1.	_____	2.	_____
4.	_____	3.	_____
7.	_____	5.	_____
9.	_____	6.	_____
10.	_____	8.	_____
11.	_____	12.	_____
14.	_____	13.	_____
18.	_____	15.	_____
19.	_____	16.	_____
23.	_____	17.	_____
24.	_____	20.	_____
26.	_____	21.	_____
27.	_____	22.	_____
29.	_____	25.	_____
30.	_____	28.	_____
31.	_____	36.	_____
32.	_____	37.	_____
33.	_____	40.	_____
34.	_____	41.	_____
35.	_____		
38.	_____		
39.	_____		

TOTAL   **A =** _____   **B =** _____

2. Add the scores in column A. This is your WHAT score.

3. Add the scores in column B. This is your WHO score.

4. Graph your WHAT and WHO scores on the following chart.

5. How to graph your WHAT and WHO scores:
   a. Put a dot on line A on the point that represents your WHAT score.
   b. Draw a line from that dot, perpendicular to line A.
   c. Put a dot on line B on the point that represents your WHO score.
   d. Draw a line from that dot, perpendicular to line B.
   e. The point where these two lines cross indicates your training profile.

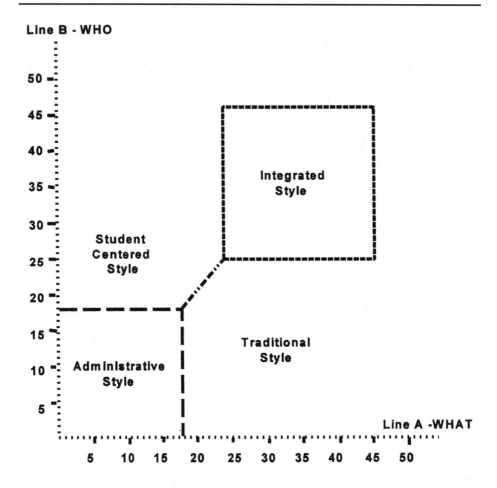

There are many ways to look at the styles of the training. This profile is designed to help you identify your training style in terms of two concerns:

■ A concern for *what* is being taught (line A).
■ A concern for *who* is being taught (line B).

These two concerns are independent variables; they can change with the subject. But most trainers have a preferred style. For example: you may have a high concern in one area and a low concern in the other, a high concern in both areas, or a low concern in both. By considering each possibility, we are able to identify four general styles, or orientations, of training.

Style Interpretations

Administrative Style

This style is characterized by low concern for both WHAT is being taught and WHO is being taught. It is essentially an "uninvolved" style of someone probably drafted against his/her will to be the practice's in-service trainer. The trainer simply passes the required information on to the other staff members, adding little of him-/herself to the presentation. Evaluation from the other staff receives minimal attention. This trainer tends to do everything by the book.

Traditional Style

This style is characterized by a high concern for WHAT is being taught and a low concern for WHO is being taught. It is essentially a "didactic process" style. Traditional-style trainers make all major decisions for the participants, decisions usually dictated by the subject being taught. These trainers often make negative assumptions about the participants, since they see themselves as the subject matter experts. They follow the academic approach of transmitting as much knowledge as possible to the participants. In the extreme, trainers with this style are seen as cold and callous.

Student-Centered Style

This style is characterized by a high concern for WHO is being taught and a low concern for WHAT is being taught. It is essentially a "warm, friendly" style. Student-centered trainers give up most of the decision-making authority to the participants since they tend to have very positive assumptions about them. This style is commonly used by trainers developing narratives for client relations, since the trainers see themselves as facilitators, helping the other staff explore options and providing whatever assistance might be needed. In the extreme, trainers with this style are seen as naive and soft by those using the traditional style.

Integrated Style

This style is characterized a high concern for both WHAT is being taught and WHO is learning. It is essentially an "involved" leadership style. Integrated-style trainers assume that the responsibility of learning is shared by themselves and the staff and generally have developed a realistic set of assumptions about the capabilities and attitude of the staff. They see the need for a balanced emphasis between the subject being shared and the interests of the staff. They believe strongly in the possibility of change and continuous quality improvement and tend to regard each staff member as a unique individual who has strengths to share.

FACT 1 In veterinary healthcare, we need to hire for attitude.

FACT 2 Leaders commit to developing the skills and knowledge needed by each staff member to support the practice activities.

FACT 3 Training, as well as hiring, should be the responsibility of the staff; the office manager, a technician, and a receptionist would be the most reasonable options for the new hiring team!

The practice leadership needs to set forth general guidelines for the 90-day probationary/introductory period (terms may vary by state) and then provide the who and when of the schedule, in writing, to the staff and doctors (see examples 1 and 2 below). At the end of 90 days, team fit (harmony) and job description competencies will be evaluated by the doctors and hiring team to determine if the candidate should be hired and, if so, at what wage.

EXAMPLE 1: Practice guidance/requirements for new staff member schedule (schedule for 90-day probationary period)

- Start person at "trainee's wage" with commitment to adjust to the "entry orientation wage" at end of the nonproductive orientation period.
- 5–10 work days—candidate is orientated to all areas (telephone, exotic care, ambulatory, surgery, lab, reception, etc.).
- 5–10 work days—candidate follows staff members doing pertinent jobs in duty area (this can be curtailed somewhat with very experienced workers).
- 5–10 work days—candidate does the work while the "doing staffer" follows (curtailment of this cycle should be only after 80 percent of the unique practice occurrences have been experienced by the new person).
- Staff trainers and doctors evaluate and recycle new person through orientation programs as needed.
- 10 work days—work solo.
- Practice owner(s), hospital veterinary medical director, and the hiring team meet to evaluate candidate's potential to join regular team as an independent solo staff member. This group sets a new wage for the balance of the introductory period, based on the performance to date and cash budget availability; this action sets the candidate on his/her new course of team development and participation.
- Practice owner(s), hospital veterinary medical director, and the hiring team commit to final hiring decision and another wage review at the 90-day point. They make decision based on competency, productivity, and team fit evaluation of the candidate's independent continuous quality improvement (CQI) efforts.

EXAMPLE 2: New team member orientation (schedule for first 10 days)

- Day 1—report to practice manager; learn to make coffee; follow the manager around when not reading the "Employee Manual and Protocols."
- Day 2—report to reception; watch morning reception and client admission activities (learn a little about where files and forms are kept).
- Day 3—report to inpatient technician; observe treatment room activities (learn a little about restraint procedures).
- Day 4—report to animal caretaker; assist animal caretaker in image and patient needs (could shift to grooming during part of the day).
- Day 5—report to outpatient technician; get "practice specialty time" with one or two doctors (learn about "special interest" capabilities).
- Day 6—report to reception on Saturday; watch client flow on a Saturday, from admission through discharge, from the reception area to waiting room to exam (watch for inefficiencies in client care).
- Day 7—report to technician and observe the laboratory in the morning; then shift to surgery; scrub in, don cap and gown, observe surgery (learn about aseptic sterile procedures).
- Day 8—follow the outpatient small animal doctors around; observe inside the exam room and hear what clients are told; report to each doctor as applicable.
- Day 9—report to key doctor(s); watch critical components of practice's healthcare delivery program in action.
- Day 10—report to practice manager; especially learn about discharges, then watch close-out procedures (learn importance of an accurate till).

a. It will be the staff trainer's responsibility to shift the orientation schedule depending on the needs of the new employee as well as the workload requirements. He/she will monitor the activities of each day, regardless of the action person so that he/she can evaluate the progress and make adjustments to future training schedules.

b. A written plan for the second (you follow the new staffer) and third phase (he/she follows you) of nonproductive orientation is also needed. The lead trainer is responsible for completing this and giving it to the doctor(s) before day 8 (the day the person spends with the doctor(s) in the exam rooms) of the first 10 days.

c. During the orientation and introductory hire period, the practice must be ready to "dehire" anyone who violates the team trust, proves ineffective after training, proves untrustworthy, or cannot adapt to the practice's standards of operation. Releasing individuals during this time is seldom grounds for unemployment (but this will vary by state). Dehiring is a courtesy to everyone ... it allows the candidate to seek a new vocational horizon more compatible to his/her work ethic and capabilities.

d. At 90 days, as established when the candidate was first employed on a probationary basis, an evaluation of two factors will determine if he/she will be hired to join the practice team. These two factors are inviolate:

- Team fit (the ability to work in harmony with all staff, doctors, and clients—this may even include community outreach for those in client relations positions).
- Competencies (meeting the requirements of the job description as measured against the job standards established at the beginning of the orientation and probationary period).

e. As discussed in the two earlier volumes of *Building the Successful Veterinary Practice,* the last two items of the job description are then added when the decision is made at 90 days to ask someone to join the regular staff of the practice:

- Meet the challenge/solve the problem—there is no such thing as "not my job," and each person has the unilateral authority to prevent problems from developing.
- See the need/make the improvement—there is no such thing as "nobody told me," and each person must be client centered and staff aware to ensure needed changes are continuously made for the harmony and quality of service of the practice operations.

f. All the above are possible if a practice accepts the resume as a screening tool but interviews each candidate for attitude with a set of open-ended questions that assess the traits, beliefs, and values. The following two interview guide examples (receptionist and technician) provide starting points for developing your own practice-specific assessment tools.

SAMPLE INTERVIEW GUIDE - RECEPTIONISTS

INTERVIEWER: _____ DATE: _____

CANDIDATE: _____

QUESTION	LISTEN FOR	RATE + or -
Please take me back to your 11th grade school year and tell me about your family, what type activities you were involved in, and your school grades. (opener - values)	ethics values detail caring	
What has been your proudest achievement? (assertive - values)	actual success selling factors	
Have you ever had to go against the system to do something you thought was right? Please share it with me. (assertive - values)	clear example	
Who has made the most significant contribution in the development of the person you are today? What was the nature of the contribution? (discerning - values)	specific person & effort	
What do you like about being in a veterinary healthcare facility? (relator)	giving caring	
How do you feel about working with extremely bright and dedicated people? What would be the benefits to you? (discerning)	positive "I fit" two-way	
What kind of relationship do you want to have with your co-workers? (relator)	giving caring	
What do you like about being a receptionist? (ego)	people representative	

QUESTION	LISTEN FOR	RATE + or -
How long do you think it will take you to become a good receptionist? (ego)	training time weeks to months	
How would you feel if a co-worker wanted to share a family concern with you? (empathy)	honored help/care	
If we decided the best way to help clients was an aggressive telephone outreach program, how would you react to such an idea? (strategist)	accept idea seek words set goals proactive	
How would you persuade reluctant phone shoppers to come in? (persuader)	find need quality care	
We hire a veterinarian that is a great doctor but poor at documenting details. How would you work with this person? (strategist)	do it for them set up template	
How do you feel about being asked to tell clients their pet has died? (empathy)	do it with training	
Why do you want to come to work for this specific practice? (believer)	serve others knows job	
Some people feel it is important to do their best rather than win or lose. Do you prefer to do the right thing or do you think a receptionist needs to do things right? (competitor)	do best to win do right thing for practice & patient client #1	
If you had only three adjectives to use to describe yourself, what would they be? (values)	honest ethical caring	

QUESTION	LISTEN FOR	RATE + or -
If you were dining at a nice restaurant with friends and one created a scene when the chicken was undercooked, how would you feel and react? (assertive)	supportive emotional take control solve issue	
How do you feel when someone questions the truth of what you have said? (assertive)	insulted emotional convincing	
What would you want to be doing if you were not a receptionist? (discerning)	inner struggle want to be one	
Some people assume they see a situation very quickly...like they were seeing it on TV...do you do this? (discerning)	big picture sensitive to feelings positives	
Would you say that you were a generous person? (relator)	emphatic yes not $ factor	
What kind of boss do you work most effectively with? (ego)	give parameters & latitude	
What are your favorite leisure time activities? (competitor)	group activity action-based	
What is your strongest value to us? (ego)	sense of worth	
You are talking to a good client and find out that the family has just entered a financial problem time. What would you do about pet care? (empathy)	consoles offers support comforts seek alternative	

QUESTION	LISTEN FOR	RATE + or -
Please describe to me your idea of a perfect pet owner. What makes this client the best? (persuader)	appeal to feelings & concerns	
What have you found to be the most effective way to change someone else's mind? (persuader)	appeal to feelings & concerns	
Some people need a well structured and planned day. How do you accomplish this? (strategist)	scheduling flexibility end results	
Do you communicate more effectively as a speaker or a writer? (relator)	needs both	
What is the most important goal which you organize in your life? (believer)	family make contribution mission	
What is the best way for you to develop your specific life goal(s)? (competitor)	achievement have some now	
Why is veterinary medicine and being a receptionist here important to you at this point in time? (believer)	helping caring action now personal goal	
You have a client that needs veterinary services immediately, but you have a concern whether the practice can really satisfy the client/patient needs. What would you do? (values)	not sell with doubts client #1 self-learning motivation	
Some people feel that anyone can be trained to be a good receptionist. How would you respond to this concept? (believer)	disagree personality caring person special skill	

QUESTION	LISTEN FOR	RATE + or -
Why should we consider you a better choice than some of the others we have interviewed? (competitor)	dedication calling capabilities	
Some receptionists want to know a great deal about the technical aspects of the profession so they can help clients. How do you feel about this? (strategist)	balance not doctor strives to know right information	
A technician feels that the front receptionist team is not screening client calls adequately. How do you respond? (persuader)	understand refer to the technical seek advice	
If I asked a previous employer what your two best attributes would be as a member of this team, what would be the reply? (believer)	voice skill empathy sensitivity dedication	

Comments: _____

_____

_____

_____

_____

_____

_____

_____

_____

PROFILE TRAITS	TOTAL +	TOTAL -
PERSUADER		
STRATEGIST		
ASSERTIVE		
EGO		
DISCERNING		
RELATOR		
EMPATHY		
VALUES		
COMPETITOR		
BELIEVER		
TOTALS		

Other Observations:

_____

_____

_____

_____

_____

_____

_____

_____

_____

_____

_____

_____

SAMPLE INTERVIEW GUIDE - TECHNICIANS

INTERVIEWER: _____ DATE: _____

CANDIDATE: _____

QUESTION	LISTEN FOR	RATE + or -
Please take me back to your 11th grade school year and tell me about your family, what type activities you were involved in, and your school grades. (opener - values)	ethics values detail caring	
What has been your proudest achievement? (assertive - values)	actual success selling factors	
Have you ever had to go against the system to do something you thought was right? Please share it with me. (assertive - values)	clear example	
Who has made the most significant contribution in the development of the person you are today? What was the nature of the contribution? (discerning - values)	specific person & effort	
What do you like about being in a veterinary healthcare facility? (relator)	giving caring	
How do you feel about working with extremely bright and dedicated people? What would be the benefits to you? (discerning)	positive "I fit" two-way	
What kind of relationship do you want to have with your co-workers? (relator)	warm friendly open	
What do you like about being a technician? (ego)	health care technical skill	

QUESTION	LISTEN FOR	RATE + or -
How long do you think it will take you to become a good receptionist? (ego)	training time weeks to months	
How would you feel if a co-worker wanted to share a family concern with you? (empathy)	honored help/care	
If we decided the best way to help clients was an aggressive telephone outreach program, how would you react to such an idea? (strategist)	accept idea seek words set goals proactive	
How would you persuade reluctant phone shoppers to come in? (persuader)	find need quality care	
We hire a veterinarian that is a great doctor but poor at documenting details. How would you work with this person? (strategist)	do it for them set up template	
How do you feel about being asked to tell clients their pet has died? (empathy)	do it with training	
Why do you want to come to work for this specific practice? (believer)	serve others knows job	
Some people feel it is important to do their best rather than win or lose. Do you prefer to do the right thing or do you think a receptionist needs to do things right? (competitor)	do best to win do right thing for practice & patient client #1	
If you had only three adjectives to use to describe yourself, what would they be? (values)	honest ethical caring	

QUESTION	LISTEN FOR	RATE + or -
If you were dining at a nice restaurant with friends and one created a scene when the chicken was undercooked, how would you feel and react? (assertive)	supportive emotional take control solve issue	
How do you feel when someone questions the truth of what you have said? (assertive)	insulted emotional convincing	
What would you want to be doing if you were not a technician? (discerning)	inner struggle want to be one	
Some people assume they see a situation very quickly...like they were seeing it on TV...do you do this? (discerning)	big picture sensitive to feelings positives	
Would you say that you were a generous person? (relator)	emphatic yes not $ factor	
What kind of team do you work most effectively with? (ego)	give parameters & latitude	
What are your favorite leisure time activities? (competitor)	group activity action-based	
What is your strongest value to us? (ego)	sense of worth	
You are talking to a good client and find out that the family has just entered a financial problem time. What would you do about pet care? (empathy)	consoles offers support comforts seek alternative	
Please describe to me your idea of a perfect pet owner. What makes this client the best? (persuader)	knows need listens steward	

QUESTION	LISTEN FOR	RATE + or -
What have you found to be the most effective way to change someone else's mind? (persuader)	appeal to feelings & concerns	
Some people need a well structured and planned day. How do you accomplish this? (strategist)	scheduling flexibility end results	
Do you communicate more effectively as a speaker or a writer? (relator)	Needs both	
What is the most important goal which you organize in your life? (believer)	family make contri- bution mission	
What is the best way for you to develop your specific life goal(s)? (competitor)	achievement have some now	
Why is veterinary medicine and being a technician here important to you at this point in time? (believer)	helping caring action now personal goal	
You have a client who needs veterinary services immediately, but you have a concern whether the practice can really satisfy the client/patient needs. What would you do? (values)	not sell with doubts client #1 self-learning motivation	
Some people feel that anyone can be trained to be a good technician. How would you respond to this concept? (believer)	disagree personality caring person special skill	
Why should we consider you a better choice than some of the others we have interviewed? (competitor)	dedication calling capabilities	

QUESTION	LISTEN FOR	RATE + or -
Some technicians want to know a great deal about the diagnostic logic for the patient's care so they can help make decisions. How do you feel about this? (strategist)	balance not doctor strives to know right information	
A receptionist feels that the back technician team is not providing them with adequate updates for when a client calls. How do you respond? (persuader)	understand find a safe method seek advice	
If I asked a previous employer what your two best attributes would be as a member of this team, what would be the reply? (believer)	voice skill empathy sensitivity dedication	

Comments: _____

_____

_____

_____

_____

_____

_____

_____

_____

_____

_____

_____

PROFILE TRAITS	TOTAL +	TOTAL -
PERSUADER		
STRATEGIST		
ASSERTIVE		
EGO		
DISCERNING		
RELATOR		
EMPATHY		
VALUES		
COMPETITOR		
BELIEVER		
TOTALS		

Other Observations:

_____

_____

_____

_____

_____

_____

_____

_____

_____

_____

_____

Build Your Own Interview

Following are questions that can be used to tailor each interview to the position for which you're hiring.

Early Background

1. Generally, how would you describe the family environment in which you were raised?

2. How would you describe your parents? What did they do for a living?

3. Do you have any brothers or sisters? Tell me about your family.

4. How do you think your family would have described you near the end of high school?

5. What aspects of growing up did you enjoy the most? The least? Why?

Education

1. What kind of student were you in high school?

2. In what extracurricular activities did you participate?

3. What kind of leadership roles did you play during your education years?

4. What honors or awards did you receive?

5. What courses did you enjoy the most? The least? Why?

6. What did you learn from your last year in school?

7. Who influenced you during your high school years?

8. What adjectives would you use to describe yourself during your most recent school years?

9. How well did your schooling prepare you for later life, in general terms?

College

1. How did you decide upon your major?

2. If you could go back in time, would you select a different major/university? Why?

3. What accounted for your grade point average?

4. Which course did you enjoy the most? The least? Why?

5. What did you do in your spare time?

6. Approximately how much time was spent studying each week? In extracurricular activities? In social activities? Why did this mix seem appropriate for your needs?

7. How did you pay for your college education?

8. Who had the greatest influence upon your direction in life during your college days?

Work Experience

1. Of the employers for whom you have worked, which did you like the most? Why?

2. Of the employers in your past, which made the work environment most distasteful? Why?

3. Of your past positions, which one did you like most? Least? Why?

4. In the various environments where you have worked, what factors made you most productive? Which ones caused decreased productivity?

5. Please compare the two environments and discuss the ways they were the same. In what ways were they different?

6. Please tell me which aspects of your past positions have best prepared you for this job.

7. In what technical areas do you feel you have the greatest strengths? Which ones need further development?

8. What specific capabilities do you feel are critical to this position?

9. What are some of the first things that you would do to make this position "yours"? Which would you save for later?

10. On a scale of 1 to 10 (10 being the highest), how would you rate your potential for successful performance in this position?

11. What circumstances led you to your last job? What factors made you decide it was the place for you?

12. What did your last job title really mean?

13. What were your functional responsibilities in the last two jobs you held?

14. What business/management/financial functions did you handle directly? Which functions were the most fun? Which functions caused you the greatest concerns?

15. What have been your major accomplishments in the workplace?

16. In what ways could your performance be improved? What steps have you taken to address these areas?

17. How would you describe your relationship with your supervisor? Your peers? Those who worked for you?

18. How do you see the job market changing over the next few years? What are you doing to prepare for these changes?

19. What aspects of your past position did you enjoy the most? Enjoy the least? Perform the best? Perform least well? Why do you say that?

20. What were the major challenges faced by your teammates?

21. What kind of performance evaluation system has worked best for you in previous employment positions? How did it work? What were the requirements for the various rating levels?

22. Which aspects of your supervisor's management philosophy worked best for the team? Which aspects had little or no effect on the performance or productivity of the team?

23. In which areas of performance was your supervisor most complimentary? Which were the areas where the most criticism fell? What did you do to react to these pro and con positions?

24. How qualified do you feel to perform the duties of this position?

Management Effectiveness

1. State your management philosophy in 25 words or less. How would you describe your management style?

2. What do you believe are characteristics of good management? Bad management?

3. What are the most effective techniques you have encountered for managing others?

4. What do you do to encourage employee freedom and participation in organizational decisions?

5. What kind of decisions should be delegated? Which ones should be retained by management?

6. What criteria should be used to measure personal performance and positional growth?

7. What managerial controls do you feel will work most of the time on most of the people?

8. What would past fellow workers say are your managerial strengths? What adjectives would they use?

9. What techniques have you found useful to motivate other people? How have you applied these skills?

10. What would you describe as the major differences between leadership and management?

11. How would you handle a team member who is handling less than his/her fair share of the work? Handling his/her share in a marginal method?

12. What do you see as the critical resources needed to get this job done effectively and efficiently?

13. How would you expect these resources to be handled to ensure profitable outcomes?

14. Which elements of the job description appear to be fuzzy, out of place, or undefinable?

15. What are your opinions concerning the elements of an effective planning cycle for this position? How do you see yourself contributing to the process?

16. How do you think the practice goals and objectives of this position should be set? Why?

17. Which are the management areas that you would like assistance and/or training in during the first year?

Personal Effectiveness

1. How would you describe your personality type? What are the strengths of that personality profile? The weaknesses?

2. If we had three of your closest work peers in this room, how would they describe your personality type under stress?

3. How do you usually handle interpersonal conflicts in the workplace? Socially? Why are they different/same?

4. If there was something you could change about yourself, what would it be? What would you want to change it to?

5. What traits, habits, or characteristics make it difficult for you when learning how to relate to someone else? In them? In you?

6. What is your most effective method to avoid conflict?

7. How would you confront someone whom you disagreed with?

8. With what aspects of your life are you most happy at this time? Least happy? Why?

9. What are your short-term career objectives? Long-term career objectives? What has been the progress in each area during the past 18 months?

10. How would you describe the potential of this position in fulfilling your career objectives?

11. How would you characterize the ideal work environment?

12. What hobbies or activities do you enjoy? How often do you participate in them? What are the rewards you feel you get from pursuing these hobbies or activities?

13. What is the level of your activity in community organizations?

14. What self-improvement plans do you have? When was the last time you pursued one of these self-improvement activities?

15. Describe the perfect job for a person with your talents and capabilities.

16. How would you compare this position with others that you have held or are pursuing?

17. What references can you supply me? Describe your relationship with each person.

18. Does you current employer know you are exploring a position move? What is/would be his/her opinion about you and this position?

19. Do you have any health problems that would impede your ability to perform within this facility and position?

20. How much advanced notice do you need to work overtime?

21. Are there any questions that you would like to ask about the facility, our practice philosophy, or the position?

22. Is there anything else you feel is important for me to know about you?

Most people who know me, and know how I approach a consultation, will tell you I do not hold a lot of value in the quick fix or gimmick. At face value this is true, but in fact, it is wrong. An integrated consultation plan is a series of gimmicks and quick fixes supported by training and sufficient explanations so the practice team can do the evaluation the next time without me. An integrated management program allows expertise to develop within the team and prepares the staff members to effectively grab opportunities before they are past, without a consultant telling them to "go for it!" As such, these 101 ideas are offered for selective integration into your practice's master plan, at the appropriate time, by the staff member responsible for the successful outcome. Integration, staff training, innovation, creativity, and forecasted programs are critical elements of success.

1. **Hydraulic lift table**—saves backs and assists in animal restraint.

2. **Ten-minute flex scheduling (e.g., ProFiles) appointment log**—variable appointment length allows more cost-effective healthcare delivery.

3. **Microchip I.D. implant**—small as a grain of rice, high tech and high touch, and an income center in itself.

4. **Tympanic temperature scanner**—measures body core temperature in seconds, is perceived by clients as high tech and high value, is OSHA compatible, and provides cost savings to practice.

5. **Something mailed to every phone shopper**—do the usual in an unusual way; booking just one extra client a day is a $25,000 annual increase in gross.

6. **Recognition of a different staff member's risk effort each day**—reward and celebrate the new mistake; starve the status quo.

7. **Mailbox of every team member**—distribute the policy and protocol in writing; only discuss the implementation ideas at staff meetings.

8. **Scrapbooks**—in a wall rack in each exam room with pet pictures, hospital tour photos, thank you notes, community accolades, and other practice pride factors.

9. **Pet adoption center**—coordinated through local Humane Society–Pet Placement Assistance (AVMA) checklists, increases traffic and new puppy/kitten access rates.

10. **Behavior management—Promise/Gentle Leader head collar**—power steering in eight minutes for most dogs (not eight weeks of obedience

school), behavior management appointments for technicians ($20/20 minute), call Ameri-Pet, 800/333-8363 (this is also the place to get the new client-centered **house training posters** for +"value-added" first puppy visit).

11. **White board in treatment**—all inpatient/day care patients recorded on board with required treatments. Anyone can write on it *but only* the senior technician can erase (after recording in medical record and tracking sheet).

12. **Lighted grooming table**—better underlighting for dermatology evaluations and grooming clips; perceived by clients as a special touch.

13. **FOR DEPOSIT ONLY**—self-inking stamp at reception for every check received, immediately stamped on back upon receipt from client.

14. **Farewell thank-you with caring message (nonsell)**—such as "drive safely," "have a happy day," etc., all in spirit of sharing "family feelings."

15. **Animal services brochure**—poison control and shelter/animal control phone numbers as well as kennel clubs, cat clubs, and other noncompetitors (e.g., an equine practitioner if you are small animal only), along with your own practice's number, provided free to realtors for distribution to newcomers researching the area.

16. **Color consistency**—among stationery, business cards, brochures, reminder cards, etc.

17. **Exit telephone surveys**—anyone who missed a final reminder gets a caring call and is asked if he/she would answer the two critical questions (what was a good memory and what was the worst experience).

18. **Promotion on hold**—short, 20-second messages, interspersed with neutral music (e.g., New Age), to educate, inform, and cross-market services.

19. **Patient data cover sheets**—color-coded by sex, with minimum wellness screen expected on recurring basis for any patient accessing the practice.

20. **All teeth graded in medical records**—1+, 2+, 3+, 4+ (e.g., CET brochure), send brochure home with client, arrow means no care is provided, crossed out arrow means technician is assigned to case.

21. **Scoreboard**—visual display entered daily, posted in staff area, on monthly item(s) of special interest, such as gross, number of fecals, callbacks, new clients, etc.

22. **Front-faced shelf items**—group by species and function, largest size to right; priced items only put on shelf if in durable multimonth packaging.

23. **Name tag**—clear and distinct on every team member (right side), with title of staff member's choosing, denoting special interest/training level.

24. **Staff brochure**—profile of each full-time staff member in a trifold to highlight his/her community involvement and practice expertise.

25. **Mystery shopper**—evaluates either by phone or office visit and is capable of recognizing superior care or neglect, objective measurement of individual and team performance.

26. **"How are we doing?" random telephone surveys of clients**—what could be improved, how can we better serve our clients, etc.?

27. **Toy box for kids, in out-of-way corner.**

28. **Medical staff picture gallery**—8×10-inch framed color pictures in waiting area, with name and short biography, as well as professional associations and degrees.

29. **Automatic X-ray processor**—faster, better pictures, client views dry films without streaks.

30. **Dental hygiene technician**—all deferred care gets technician assigned, and technician does monthly courtesy rechecks for "red means pain."

31. **Human interest bulletin board (refrigerator magnet)**—just-for-fun cartoons, newspaper articles, humorous stories, baby pictures, birthdays, etc.

32. **Client emotions appealed to, not professional logic**—allow clients to "buy" to meet their emotional needs; do not "sell" just because it is logical.

33. **Coordinated uniform colors**—image consistency, with logo, to give impression of coordinated team effort and image of quality.

34. **Pet health records**—issued or updated with vaccines or other recurring wellness care.

35. **DEA checklist**—system to allow different individuals to spot-check the controlled substance security and tracking systems.

36. **Courtesy checklist "report cards"**—(5×8-inch max) for boarders being discharged so client knows next needs (and can keep list on refrigerator).

37. **Clients referring five new clients in a year get a brass plate recognition**—permanent plaque in reception area (plus or minus the permanent 10 percent preferred client recognition discount).

38. **Picture tour "behind the scenes" in reception**—labeled with who is doing what to which animal.

39. **Dry chemistry machine**—to support presurgical screens (consent forms with laboratory test waiver).

40. **Receptionist new client luncheon**—any month when over 60 percent of new clients have come by word-of-mouth referral, receptionists are taken out by "Doc" for a celebration lunch (technicians staff the front desk).

41. **Competition vital signs**—break room bulletin board on community and vicinity veterinary offerings by competition.

42. **Price-sensitive items**—know price-sensitive items (e.g., vaccines, food, insecticides) versus unknown commodity items (e.g., collars, Nylabones, etc.) and price accordingly.

43. **Medical rounds**—early morning (before any appointments) walk-through doctor review with kennel caretakers and senior technicians to check overnight changes and coming day needs of each patient.

44. **Clearly annotated "sorry we inconvenienced you" premium**—(e.g., ice cream coupon) awarded when practice ineffectiveness delays client (late appointment) or has added a hassle factor.

45. **Plastic sleeves for pet health records**—adds importance and a do-not-discard impression for clients.

46. **Incidence map**—community map in reception with pins showing each animal's location with incidence of specific disease (heartworm, FeLV, etc.).

47. **VCR in each exam room**—offer a selection of tapes; keep list on new client information form to prevent duplication.

48. **New patient Polaroid photo board in reception.**

49. **IV pump**—measured fluid therapy system.

50. **Animal's weight recorded in the medical records at every visit**—10 percent weight changes get technician assigned to follow the case monthly.

51. **Contest of the month**—internal practice emphasis on exceeding previous set target with known staff dividend for exceeding expectation (dinner, $, etc.).

52. **Drive through pneumatic tube system**—for refill prescriptions and curbside service to elderly, handicapped, clients with kids in car, no make-up, etc.

53. **For boarding activities, boarders are "guests" and cages or runs are "suites" or "habitats" or "play areas."**

54. **Video-lending library**—at no cost, for established clients.

55. **Thank-you for the referral letters**—with another brochure for the next client they want to send.

56. **OSHA checklist**—allows different staff members to spot-check the practice for safety hazards and protection programs. This should include the OSHA warning signs—have these available for slippery floors, dangerous animals, heavy loads, chemical hazards, and other liability precautions.

57. **Information literature rack**—ensure no client departs without something relevant in hand.

58. **Clean and clear reception counter**—displays and ads belong in retail or on wall shelves, not reception counter.

59. **X-ray view box in each exam room**.

60. **Nutritional counselor**—each nutritional case gets courtesy monthly weigh-in and/or technician follow-up until condition is resolved.

61. **Smile mirror between back room and front with simple note—"How will clients see you today?"**

62. **Emergency stickers**—front door or window sticker to alert firefighters there are pets inside, a constant daily reminder to client of practice's concern.

63. **No-strings-attached premium**—(e.g., two movie tickets, two zoo tickets, etc.) for "thank you for *another* referral" letter (merchant booklets available at discount rates from most multiplex theatres); this is also tax deductible—practice discounts are not.

64. **Medical record checklist**—allows anyone to do peer review for essential elements of wellness care documented in patient records.

65. **Coat rack/umbrella stand**—clients prefer a safe place to put these things where animals will not soil them.

66. **Museum**—heartworm display (704/584-0381), old instruments, kidney stones, flea under a magnifying glass, etc., interspersed among the retail stock to draw client attention.

67. **Dog treat/owner treat**—thank you sheet to denote clean exam room and start encounter on positive note.

68. **Upgrade of practice sign**—injection molded and back lit, digital time and temperature updates if on busy street.

69. **Community youth programs, school speaking, facility tours, annual Scout-organized rabies vaccination clinics.**

70. **Percent appointment log fill**—any day over 80 percent fill gets receptionist's a recognition percentage of excess earning for end-of-month performance pay.

71. **New puppy/kitten checklist**—the dozen essential elements that every client with a new pet needs to hear every time.

72. **Coloring sheets**—children distracting, take home, family friendly, educational, warm and fuzzy.

73. **Client bulletin board for lost and found animals.**

74. **Personalized courtesy leashes.**

75. **Courtesy refreshments**—within reception area, client friendly refreshments available (coffee, tea, ice water, candy, etc.)

76. **Landscaping**—include pet comfort station in route between parking and facility entrance.

77. **Tattoo identification**—offered with spay and neuter procedures at reduced cost.

78. **Senior citizen large print handouts, coupled with extra appointment time.**

79. **Plexiglass cat cozy box**—with matching piano-hinged lid, in waiting area for scaredy cats.

80. **Parasite prevention and control technician**—all parasite cases get

technician assigned for return courtesy evaluation to ensure animal is free of parasites.

81. **Maintenance board**—framed list in hallway with equipment/service action, maintenance frequency, next due date, person responsible, and vendor cross-reference for outside support.

82. **Flat computer screen on consult room wall to show computerized diagnostic images.**

83. **Courtesy phone**—in reception waiting area for client use, sign above it stating it is *reserved* for client use.

84. **"Parasites of Our Community" information sheets for new clients.**

85. **Quality assurance checklists**—spot-check systems for technical aspects of facility or operational effectiveness, permitting anyone to evaluate the compliance to practice standards.

86. **Breeder registry**—list of people with purebred animals for whom they may want a mating or want to produce offspring in the future.

87. **Directional and information signs**—graphically compatible with practice image.

88. **Discharge instructions**—establish both home care needs and expectation for next visit.

89. **Council of Clients**—a dozen community members brought together quarterly for dessert to act as focus group to help practice determine how to better meet client needs in the community (group can change each time).

90. **Inventory control team**—when technician team maintains inventory below desired cost of goods sold, members share percentage of quarterly savings.

91. **Check stamp**—extra after-sale client service, practice name stamped on client checks to save writing facility name.

92. **Custom carriers**—with practice name/logo, sold at cost, as client service plus name recognition.

93. **New client newsletter**—seldom changes, profiles the practice and the key staff and doctors, shares beliefs and describes common surgical procedure and special programs.

94. **Client relations specialist**—unilateral solver of client problems, "What can we do to make it right?"

95. **Practice hours posted**—easily read from inside a car in the parking lot (including lighting at night).

96. **Feline-friendly cat health month.**

97. **Respiratory monitor**—audio monitoring from trach tube, set with rate alarm, for secondary protection.

98. **Two-headed microscope or TV attachment for client education via monitor.**

99. **Timers on back of exam rooms**—to ensure timely client service, coupled with colored flags (lights) to call attention to next need in exam room.

100. **Pet tag display**—better patient ID, information to save pet's life, profits can go to practice party fund.

101. **Empowered staff**—to solve problems, add innovations, and meet client needs, without permission or direction.

So now, get out there, offer that vaccination warranty you read about in *Veterinary Economics* (oops, gimmick number 102), and have fun integrating your programs.

Definition

Computerized medical records are based on a relational database where a *single medical record entry* drives multiple retrieval systems, from inventory adjustments and invoicing to prescriptions and treatment plans.

Reality Test

If this relational database system really exists, we could do the following query (although it may require multiple queries to get the classifications delineated, the original input would be from the single-entry progress notes):

Retrieve all bilateral canine otitis externa cases seen in the past eight months, compare treatment results and return rates for those treated with (1) Panalog, (2) Tresaderm, (3) Mitox, or (4) Otomax, and show the average total cost and average client transaction income associated with each treatment modality.

POMR

The problem-oriented medical record (POMR) format is the standard in veterinary medical records. It is based on four elements: subjective (history), objective (exam), assessment (what we are treating), and plan (here is what we can do); thus, the terminology SOAP or HEAP is used when talking about appropriate medical record annotations. The assessment (of HEAP or SOAP) takes many forms, each meaning something slightly different in a court of law:

- A = assessment = this is what the above (HE or SO) means to me.
- Dx = tentative diagnosis = the most probable cause.
- Ddx = differential diagnosis = these are all the possible causes of the signs we are seeing.
- R/O = rule out = the treatment plan below will either rule out the signs (or this best guess disease) or rule out the treatment.
- Observation: from the above discussion, it is evident that, forensically, R/O is the safest and is, in fact, the only one that has not yet been litigated to the detriment of the healthcare provider.

Problems

The POMR is based on identifying problems, but in fact, veterinarians often treat probabilities rather than use diagnostics. More importantly, today we are treating wellness, not problems. Vol. 2 provides a foundation for this concept, with forms and formats, so please review it if you have any questions. Depending on the diagnostic ability of the practice, about 10 to 30 percent of the cases return unresolved, which requires a change in therapy. As such, each assessment (R/O, Dx, Ddx, etc.) needs to be numbered and listed in a master problem list if it is to be followed at a later date. *An assessment that is open means symptomatic care is being offered*—ensure that medical logic is stated clearly! The number precludes reiteration of the SOA and HEA portion of the medical record entry and allows the provider to go directly to the new/revised/modified treatment plan.

Rationale

While the computer has become the primary client relations tool, the medical record needs to be the cornerstone of continuity of patient care, whether the information is recorded on computer or paper. The invoicing and reminders, while critical to the business of veterinary practice, are secondary to this healthcare requirement. There are certain critical elements of information that *must be written, legibly,* in the progress notes of the medical records (please review Chapter 1, *AAHA Standards for the Accreditation of Veterinary Hospitals*):

• Patient-specific medical records (client-patient)
• Date of presentation
• Client concerns (chief complaint) at presentation
• Abnormal history and physical exam findings
• Assessment of problem(s) (Dx, Ddx, A, R/O, etc.)
• Doctor's treatment plan
• Client's acceptance, waiver, or deferral of each element
• Diagnostics conducted with results
• Medication/prescriptions (with full SIG)
• Return/recheck/reminder/recall expectations

Discussion

The above could be streamlined, but liability would increase with deletion of critical information. The goal is not to enter the least data possible but to ensure prompts and formats accelerate the keystroke requirements for entering essential medical information. Client concern drives the examination protocol and diagnostic tests. The newer Windows-based systems have direct download of diagnostic results from the optical scanner or diagnostic machine into the patient record, and the record is retrievable in many formats, including colored graphics and merged files with photos and client instructions. The case assessment drives the treatment plan and dispensing actions. Follow-up expectations, as well as client waivers, deferrals, and acceptances, reflect the official veterinary medical agreements made with the steward of the animal for healthcare treatment of the patient. *Soon all of this will be driven from a touch screen examination room computer station.* Do not accept less. Demand the Windows upgrades from your vendor; be ready to change computer vendors if they cling to the past. The veterinary computer and software systems are changing so quickly that reputable vendors have developed a three-year plan for total conversion of all veterinary users to Windows.

Review of a Computer Vendor's Presentation

EDP Theory

The electronic data-processing (EDP) programmers usually do it backwards. The first goal should be to meet the healthcare delivery standards of the veterinary profession while working within the framework of established quality criteria (e.g., *AAHA Standards for the Accreditation of Veterinary Hospitals,* Section 1). Automation goals of most vendors are focused on the money: they start at the end—the invoice. In fact, most traditional veterinary computer systems are not much more than cash register programs linked to word processing with a mail merge capability (e.g., the Access Bible has the Mountaineer Veterinary Clinic on its demonstration disc). Look closely, very few have any ability to merge income data with expense data to drive a balance sheet and profit and loss statement, the two minimum EDP reports of any business.

Procedures

Hope you are not irate yet, please accept the fact that the industry standards are set by the American Animal Hospital Association (AAHA) and the universities; they are modified by the American Veterinary Medical Association (AVMA) trust agents who settle medical record litigation out of court.

Main System

Look at what is tracked, versus what is visually presented, when assessing the computer vendor's presentation. Graphics, or bells and whistles are nice, but they don't give you critical medical or business management information.

a. Presenting signs (client concerns)
b. New or existing client
c. New or existing patient (plus other pet screen for household)
d. New or existing sign/concern
e. Ancillary wellness needs (vaccines, heartworm, FeLV, etc.)*
f. History
g. Examination (+/ diagnostic testing)*
h. Case assessment (what are we going to treat for?)
i. Supplemental testing needs*
j. Automatic filing of testing reports into medical record*
k. Medications (full SIG)* and treatments*
l. Dispensing*/prescribing action (full SIG)
m. Automatic inventory adjustments
n. Client education
o. Next visit expectation (telephone and mail expectations, too)

Denotes a potential invoicing linkage requirement.

Consider

The hierarchy of data as proposed by most computer vendors skips most of the above steps. Veterinarians who want to retain their active licensure in practice cannot skip these. Letter h may be the master problem, or it might be a commitment to treat symptomatically if the client waived the diagnostic plan. Flexibility will be critical at this juncture.

The new visit template must be user friendly. Most veterinarians examine an animal from nose to tail and from the outside inward (compare A with B below).

A. Factors of the typical exam

Temperature, pulse, respiration rate
Weight
Coat and skin
Eyes
Ears
Nose and throat
Mouth, teeth, gums
Legs and paws
Lymph nodes
Heart
Lungs
Abdomen
Gastrointestinal
Urogenital
Anal sacs
Diet
Vaccines
Heartworm/FeLV
Fecal
External parasites
Behavior

B. Pitfalls of the traditional veterinary computer system

General appearance is emphasized more than weight and condition: bright, alert, and responsive (BAR) are three typically abused veterinary medical record entries.

Integument is skin but has often been confused with hair coat condition or ectoparasite describers.

Musculoskeletal is most often presented as pathology or trauma but has often been confused with primary locomotion describers in the program(s).

Circulatory is more than a pulse rate, mucous membranes, or capillary refill rates, but some vendors have made it only a cardiac evaluation by the describers available.

Respiratory starts at the nares and has a normal rate, but it is often restricted to the lungs by the computer template describers.

Digestive is the center of an anatomical donut, but signs such as vomiting have often been entered in the computer describers, as well as appetite (diet) and bladder (urogenital).

Genitourinary (urogenital) is the genital and urinary apparatus, but behavior has been shown as describers for genitourinary by some computer programs.

Eyes (unilateral or bilateral) most often have a discharge, are inflamed, or itch. These signs are usually missing from describers in programs.

Ears, like eyes, come in R and L and often need to go beyond the computer describers to include common conditions like itchy, inflamed, excessive hair, etc.

Neural is reflex and consciousness, but not generally behavior, although some computer describers indicate to the contrary (why would gait—a reflex—be musculoskeletal and housebreaking—a behavior—be urogenital, while behavior disposition is neural?)

Lymph nodes are found in areas other than the neck, although some programmers seem to have missed this fact.

Mucous membranes are usually evaluated in the eye and mouth, so why list them in multiple other body systems?

Disclaimer: I am not picking on any one computer vendor, but you need something a bit more innovative and creative than what has been provided. If you want to attract the quality patients to your new system, stick to paper until the computer database becomes relational (see below).

C. The emerging Windows-based veterinary computer systems:

- Ultrasound download directly into the patient record, with an "organ screen" offered as a presurgical procedure (<$50).
- Video ophthalmoscopes and episcopes recorded directly into the patient record, with matched pictures provided at recheck.
- Lead 2 screening ECG (<$20), with direct feed into the patient's medical record, and/or a physical exam digital ECG system, with contact electrodes, which will download an ECG with every outpatient physical (about $1 extra per doctor's consultation—no longer called an exam or office call).
- Fiberendoscopes with video processor and light source, to allow direct recording of highly graphical photo observations into the patient's medical records.
- Video Vetscopes, which allow the provider to a perform dental exam, ear exam, biopsies, irrigation, suction, foreign material removal, or similar procedure while under constant EDP visualization, which is automatically stored in the patient record.
- Bar-coding control of inventory, blood bank resources, equipment, and other important assets.

- Integrated time clock to payroll system, with other human resource management factors (e.g., accrued personal time).
- Tailorable appointment schedules for specialists, boarding, grooming, as well as the routine clinical functions.
- Relational database search capabilities of medical records, likely in a series of single-question eliminators or groupings, which can be programmed and searched by on-site staff, according to client location, diagnostic code, master problem list, species, age, therapy regimen, or similar practice-specific variables.
- Simplified download capabilities of income data to common spreadsheets for comparison with associated line-item expense data for the same period.
- Automatic uplink capabilities for Internet access, including veterinary information networks, systems, and libraries.

The Horizon

Is there a 32-bit, Windows-based system technology emerging in veterinary software? Are there human healthcare software vendors starting to enter the veterinary medicine software field with better developed medical record systems? Are we beginning to see vendor consolidation and sweeping improvements rather than just software gimmicks? Yes: we already are experiencing a revolution in innovativeness and creativity in veterinary software.

The audit of active medical records within the veterinary practice has traditionally been done by exception; that is, when a veterinary practice gets a complaint or asks for help on a difficult case. Here is a set of tools I developed to allow the medical record audit to become a management tool.

The Instruments

The Count Sheet

This is simply a method to keep track of your progress through 100 client records. Note I wrote "client records." When you use 100, the data automatically convert to percentages, which allow ready comparability to American Animal Hospital Association (AAHA), American Veterinary Medical Association (AVMA), or other published data. Statistical sampling may indicate that you should pull records from the ——10 to ——19 terminal digits until you get 100, but we have found that 50 or 100 consecutive records work just as well for the medical record audit.

The Client Profile

Data for the client profile come from the new client information sheet or a quick scan of the medical record for the patient mix. If you are not collecting this information, use only what you have available—do not estimate or guess. This is a "counting audit," not an ego boost. Just place a hash mark in each section as you review each client record. To use these data, you may have to do further computations. For instance, the percentage of dog households with cats has been reported by the AVMA as about 40 percent, but to compute your practice's percentage, you must divide the cat and dog households in the "Other Pets in Household" section by the total of the hash marks from one-dog, multiple-dog, and cat and dog households.

The Medical Record Assessment for Patient Advocacy

This information comes from *every* patient record in the 100 client records. It includes the partially completed records, the records that haven't been purged or annotated, and any other patient indicator in the record system. Again it is strictly a "count-it audit," not a place to estimate or guess. Just place a hash mark in each section as you review each patient's record. The computations for this section will be based on the total number of patients counted (expected to be about 164 pets per 100 households by the AVMA studies), so percentages will not be as easy to compute initially.

- As the patient records are reviewed, look for the flow of the cases, the recurrence of the problems, and especially the *plan*—the need (see Vol. 2, pp. 72–79), the client's response (W-D-A-X per Vol. 2), and the next contact expectation by the provider (three *R*s per Vol. 2).
- Besides comparing your data with the most recent AVMA study or other published trends, you can evaluate your internal marketing to some extent. By comparing the percentage of patients in the vaccination status lines of the "First-Visit Evaluation" section with the percentage of patients in the waived and current lines of the "Past Due for Vaccination" section, you can see the patient advocacy or deterioration trends affecting the services you have been offering.
- This medical record audit data can also be used when assessing the fiscal charts and marketing information. When used in conjunction with the other instruments, the cause-and-effect relationships become more apparent.

The Count Sheet

The data available from the AVMA, AAHA, *Veterinary Economics,* and other management publications are generally given in percentages. To make this charting system easier to operate, we suggest that 100 client records be used. Ensure all patients that belong to each of the 100 clients are included in the record pull. As you select a client record, record the sequential number of client records reviewed (cross out as completed).

1, 2, 3, 4, 5,	6, 7, 8, 9, 10,	11, 12, 13, 14, 15,	16, 17, 18, 19, 20,
21, 22, 23, 24, 25,	26, 27, 28, 29, 30,	31, 32, 33, 34, 35,	36, 37, 38, 39, 40,
41, 42, 43, 44, 45,	46, 47, 48, 49, 50,	51, 52, 53, 54, 55,	56, 57, 58, 59, 60,
61, 62, 63, 64, 65,	66, 67, 68, 69, 70,	71, 72, 73, 74, 75,	76, 77, 78, 79, 80,
81, 82, 83, 84, 85,	86, 87, 88, 89, 90,	91, 92, 93, 94, 95,	96, 97, 98, 99, 100

COMMENTS

By pulling 100 client records, you have a 100 percent client number for assessing the pets per household, pet mix, or similar parameters.

The patient data comparisons will require a separate math assessment for internal comparisons.

QUICK CLIENT LOYALTY ASSESSMENT

Count the total number of clients within the "S" file: _____(a)
Count those "Ss" that haven't been in during the last FY: _____(b)
Subtract (b) from (a) to get active clients in FY: $a - b =$ _____(c)
"S" is 10% of client base in the USA, so multiply by 10: $c \times 10 =$ _____(d)
Count the rabies tags (certificates) for the last FY: _____(e)
Divide (e) by (d) to get client response rate to reminders: _____%

If there are large amounts of new or walk-in clients, compute their percentage of the active client base (c) and then subtract from the above percentage to get an adjusted client loyalty impression.

The Client Profile

This database should be annually retrieved from 100 new client information sheets.*

Pick one in each category.

INCOME TYPE *(unknown**)*
    Dual income:
    One income:
    No income (retired):

SOURCE OF CLIENT *(unknown**)*
    Referral (person thanked):
    Referral (source unknown):
    Sign (drive by):
    Yellow Pages for location:
    Yellow Pages for services:

HUMAN/ANIMAL BOND *(unknown**)*
    Pet is member of family:
    Pet is just a pet:
    Single-visit client:

OTHER PETS IN HOUSEHOLD *(unknown**)*
    One cat only household:
    Multiple-cat household:
    One dog only household:
    Multiple-dog household:
    Cat and dog household:

OTHER PETS (can check more than one)
    Pet bird present:
    Pet reptile present:
    Caged mammal present:

*For example, see "Welcome to Our Practice!!" in this appendix.
**"Unknown" is used during the count to identify data not captured from appropriate data.

The Medical Record Assessment for Patient Advocacy

FIRST-VISIT EVALUATION (pick one)
    Shots PLUS fecal, FeLV, or heartworm status recorded:
    Shots w/o fecal, FeLV, or heartworm status recorded:
    Medical case without vaccination history or fecal:
    Over-the-counter sale/boarding without animal history:

PAST DUE FOR VACCINATION (pick one)
    Less than 3 months:
    More than 3 months:
    Dead or waived by client:
    Status current:

TIME SINCE LAST VISIT (pick one)
    Less than 6 months:
    6–12 months:
    12–18 months:
    18–24 months:
    Over 24 months:

OTHER CLIENT BONDING FACTORS (can check more than one)
    Single-visit patient:
    Telephone follow-up missing:
    Folder not marked with current data:
    Forms not used as designed:
    Client complaint unclear:
    Case assessment missing:
    Other pets missed:
    Client waiver/deferral/refusal entered:

WELCOME TO OUR PRACTICE ! !

Thank you for giving us the opportunity to care for your pet. Please help us meet your needs better by taking a moment to share some important information we will need as we support your pet's needs today and in the future. **PLEASE PRINT IN ALL SPACES.**

CLIENT'S NAME _____ SPOUSE/OTHER _____

ADDRESS _____ CITY _____ STATE _____ ZIP _____

CHILDREN & VISITOR NAMES _____

HOME PHONE _____ HOME FAX _____ SOC. SEC. # _____

EMPLOYER _____ WORK PHONE _____

SPOUSE/OTHER EMPLOYER _____ WORK PHONE _____

At what time (_____) and at what phone number (_____) can we call to talk to you about your pet?

Who would we ask for? _____ Alternate Emergency Number _____

We will gladly prepare a written estimate if you desire (please ask our doctor OR receptionist). This will be important to you since *ALL PROFESSIONAL FEES ARE DUE AT THE TIME SERVICES ARE RENDERED. In cases of extensive medical or surgical procedures, when full payment may be difficult at discharge, we take Master Card, Visa, or can establish a payment arrangement if approved in advance of the treatment.* There will be a $25.00 service charge for any check returned unpaid.

To prevent the spread of infectious diseases, all hospitalized and boarded patients must be current on all vaccines and free from internal and external parasites. The signature below authorizes this level of preventive care and the appropriate charges will be assessed in the discharge invoice.

Signature of Responsible Agent for Pet(s) _____ Date _____

How/Why Did You Select Us? _____

Would You Like Behavior Management Assistance? _____

Have your pet(s) traveled out of the area? Where? _____

ESSENTIAL PET INFORMATION

PET'S NAME	SPECIES	DATE OF BIRTH	SEX	S/N	DESCRIPTION

COMMUNITY CHARACTERISTICS

Catchment Area (80% client pull) Characteristic	Today	5 Years Ago
Area Economy (strong, stable, recessionary, etc.)		
Number of Active Client Records (Active = ___year cull interval)		
Average Family Income in Catchment Area (in "___,000")		
Total Annual County Community Income (in millions$)		
➤ Three-Mile Radius Catchment Area Income (in millions$)		
➤ Five-Mile Radius Catchment Area Income (in millions$)		
Percent Single Unit Dwellings within 20 minutes		
Education Level in Primary Catchment Area		
Community Identity (High, Moderate, Low, Walled Subdivisions)		
Percent Dual Income Families		
Crime Level in Area (High, Moderate, Low)		
Percent Patients That Are Dogs		
Percent Patients That Are Avian/Exotics		
Percent Senior Citizens		
Percent Breeders		
Percent Clients Bringing Kids		
Total Hours of Evenings (after 6:00 p.m.)/Weekend Access		
➤ Evening Hours		
➤ Weekend Hours		
Drop-Off Patients Per Week		
Percent Appointments Filled (total appointment hours/week:_____)		
Number of Other Practices within 5 Minutes		
Number of Other Practices within 20 Minutes		
Number of Boarding Kennels within 20 Minutes		
Number of Pet Supply Stores within 20 Minutes		

Repositionable Puzzles

There are two ways to be remembered in the marketplace and in life:

■ Do the usual as if it were unusual.
■ Do the unusual as if it were usual.

A company called Abilities Unlimited (303-773-2332) introduced me to "repositionable puzzles," which have a major benefit for individual practice tailoring (cost of 5,000 sheets is $0.28 for the 5x8-inch puzzle in one color). The concept is illustrated below:

				Fleas can carry	A female cat is called a	An injection to protect an animal from rabies is called an
Lyme Disease	technician	six		_____	_____	_____
tapeworms	queen	seven		All pets deserve a _____	Baby goats are called _____	Animals need water _____
immunization	kids	pet!		Mosquitos can bite a dog and give it _____.	A veterinary doctor has ____ or more years of college.	Ticks can cause a disease called _____ in people.
women	heartworms	all the time		Most of the new graduate veterinarians are _____	One year of a dogs life is about equal to ____ people years.	A veterinary nurse is often called a veterinary _____

As you can see, the shaded area on the left has sticker squares containing answers, which can be placed over the statements on the right to complete them (you can make up your own statements). The unique aspect is that the shaded squares will form the graphic of your choice when assembled atop the correct squares. The graphic can be printed at no additional cost when provided as camera ready art. Just think of the pictures you could make!

The Preferred Client Program
An Alternative to Discount Coupons

Vol. 2 presents a narrative that was used for a 10-minute vaccination appointment, without an annual doctor's consultation, for "good clients" who see the veterinarian every three to four months. However, 75 percent of these good clients still wanted to see the doctor! The **preferred client program** is a more extensive service for communities with great competition or multiple levels of veterinary health care advertised in the media.

Concept

Preferred clients are defined as those who keep their pets fully protected (for all elements of the pink [♀] or blue [♂] patient data cover sheet, Vol. 2)—allowing nothing to expire. Staff can readily identify these by a color-coded screen on the computer as well as through the patient data sheet.

Benefit

Preferred clients get commodity healthcare items at rates competitive with the local Humane Society (about $2 above for each wellness item it quotes on the phone)—by the outpatient nursing staff in most cases (some states have restrictions)—*but* the doctor's consultation is always offered as an option with any outpatient nurse appointment, with a narrative similar to the Vol. 2 narrative discussed above (and we will see greater than a 75 percent optional doctor consultation access rate in most client-bonding practices when the narrative is smooth).

Reason

The front door must swing! If the clients are driven out of the practice, nothing can be provided. Every client contact is an opportunity to screen all the pets of the household for wellness so the client can access less expensive veterinary health care while protecting their pets (who are family members). And the staff can really buy into this concept.

Belief

If veterinarians are the stewards of animal wellness in the community, we need to be the champions all of the time. The days of veterinary practices living off inflated income from vaccines and volume-based surgical sterilization are coming to an end. These products are becoming commodities that will readily be available to all. Today, medicine and surgery must carry the veterinary practice. New technologies will allow diagnostics to be directly entered into the computer, will give clients a visual look inside the science of veterinary medicine, but, more importantly, will become the key differentiating factors between practices.

Secret

The power lies in the staff's belief systems, which are founded on the core values of the practice. The leader who establishes this type of program will see the staff rally around it to promote wellness like never before. This is a program that targets the beliefs of staff, the wants of clients, and the needs of the patients. It is a true veterinary stewardship program for clients who care.

Each of the statements below corresponds to common coping methods. For each statement, circle the number that most clearly corresponds to how frequently you act that way in a difficult situation. Then total your scores for each section.

	often	sometimes	rarely	never
1. I go to sleep when things get bad.	3	2	1	0
2. I don't get involved in problems.	3	2	1	0
3. I forget important facts.	3	2	1	0
4. I do anything to avoid facing major tasks.	3	2	1	0
5. I never get mentally into what I have to do.	3	2	1	0
6. I don't plan ahead.	3	2	1	0
7. I forget about difficult things I have to face.	3	2	1	0
8. I am cautious and shy away from risks.	3	2	1	0
9. I avoid challenges.	3	2	1	0
SUBTOTAL	___	___	___	___
10. I never like to express my feelings.	3	2	1	0
11. When I'm upset, I tend to keep it in.	3	2	1	0
12. I get frustrated.	3	2	1	0
13. I go off alone when I get upset.	3	2	1	0
14. I try not to argue even if I feel that I want to.	3	2	1	0
15. I prepare myself for pressure and plan.	3	2	1	0
SUBTOTAL	___	___	___	___
16. I often blame others for my problems.	3	2	1	0
17. I blow up.	3	2	1	0
18. I feel irritable.	3	2	1	0
19. I cry if I lose control.	3	2	1	0
20. I know when I feel angry.	3	2	1	0
SUBTOTAL	___	___	___	___
21. I can't do one thing without thinking of two more things that I should be doing.	3	2	1	0
22. I don't recognize my achievements.	3	2	1	0
23. I put others before myself.	3	2	1	0
24. I rarely have time for myself.	3	2	1	0
25. I worry about things.	3	2	1	0
26. I don't have time for hobbies.	3	2	1	0
27. I like to do everything myself.	3	2	1	0
28. I feel impatient if I have to wait.	3	2	1	0
29. I'm rushed on most things.	3	2	1	0
30. I try to be on time for everything.	3	2	1	0
SUBTOTAL	___	___	___	___
GRAND TOTAL	___	___	___	___

Understanding Your Profile

Numbers 1–9 are withdrawal characteristics, numbers 10–15 are internalizing characteristics, numbers 16–20 are outburst characteristics, and numbers 21–30 are control characteristics.

Withdrawal

If your score was high in areas 1–9, you are not meeting your responsibilities, and you are holding back from life. This can lead to worry, anger, and frustration.

Things to do to change:

1. Visualize yourself completing what you want done and feel the benefits.

2. Give yourself rewards for things you complete; a good feeling can defuse the hidden anger and frustration.

3. Take small steps toward expressing yourself.

4. Make a list of things you need and want to do; assign dates for starting and completing each item.

5. List your fears but include the rewards for overcoming the fears.

6. Think about how you felt the last time you didn't do what you needed to do (the anger, frustration, depression); then think about all the reasons you don't want to feel this way again and get started.

Internalizing

If your score was high in areas 10–15, you are building resentment and anger while shutting out those who care about you. You are probably causing yourself a great deal of internal stress in an attempt to relieve the daily pressure(s).

Things to do to change:

1. Write down some reasons for why you should not share your feelings; then look at them as someone who cares about a person who has those reasons.

2. Separate your feelings from the demands you're making on yourself.

3. Understand that you can express yourself without anyone else being obligated to do something about it.

4. Don't speculate about what others will think.

Outbursts

If your score was high in areas 16–20, you may be internalizing feelings of helplessness. Shifting blame and responsibility for outbursts is a self-defeating response to frustration or anger. This is passing on the anger and frustration, not resolving the pressure(s).

Things to do to change:

1. Become aware of the emotions that trigger the outbursts; your "shoulds" can cause distress from childhood on.

2. If "life" causes the emotions, take it as a signal for creativity and change.

3. Ask yourself why you feel the way you do; look for the cause in the past, even the far past.

4. Seek other ways to better express yourself, especially if you can recenter on a better self-esteem and image.

Control

If your score was high in areas 21–30, your behavior is probably Type A—you try to control every situation and to plan for every possible problem. Trying to keep control over your world is unrealistic and creates anger and anxiety. You become tired and frustrated taking care of everything around you.

Things to do to change:

1. Evaluate all priorities and tasks. Ensure you have allocated tasks to at least three separate categories: (1) do immediately, (2) do after the immediate, and (3) only start after the first two categories are depleted.

2. Confront the fear of not being in control; shift from the need for control to clearly identifying the desired outcomes and letting others determine the process.

3. Look honestly at the beliefs and feelings that are behind your behavior; anger and fear will not get what you want.

General Thoughts to Add to Your Self-Assessment

1. Ask yourself, "Just how long do I intend to be miserable?" You can manage your feelings.

2. In stressful times, you have the right to feel frustrated, angry, and depressed; you also have the right to change your feelings to positive thoughts.

3. If others don't live up to your expectations, change your expectations: turn to creative and innovative assistance programs.

4. Don't berate yourself; assume responsibility for your actions and pursue a more productive and joyous life.

This appendix offers ideas and methods, icebreakers and exercises, that will allow a caring leader to create a better environment for innovation and creativity.

Team Creativity Exercise 1
Doublespeak

The Doublespeak of the Would Be Leader

1. Should an evolutional eohippus entity be made available to you without expectation of remuneration, refrain from making an ocular foray into the oral cavity of that entity.

2. Deleterious consequences often precipitate from accelerated execution.

3. Do not traverse an edifice erected to afford passage over an abyssal void until the temporal eventually is imminent.

4. Sagacity dictates that one not excise the proboscis as a punitive measure against one's personal visage.

5. It is not advantageous to garner the totality of one's gallinaceous collections into a singular receptacle made of compliant twigs.

6. Lexical truncations, abbreviations, or similar condensations can be equated to the quintessence or very spiritual embodiment of persiflage.

Match terms to meanings:

1. Safety-related occurrence	a. To taste or smell something
2. Incomplete success	b. The poor
3. Fiscal underachievers	c. Pigpens and chicken coops
4. Small animal repairman	d. Thermometer
5. Non–goal-oriented member of society	e. Bank robbery
6. Single-purpose agricultural structure	f. Newspaper delivery person
7. Downsizing personnel	g. Accident
8. Advanced downward adjustments	h. Budget cuts
9. Collateral damage	i. Frightened
10. Ultimate high-intensity warfare	j. Street person
11. Media courier	k. Antisatellite weapons
12. Unauthorized withdrawal	l. Failure
13. Digital fever computer	m. Veterinarian
14. Conduct an organoleptic analysis	n. Civilian casualties of war
15. Philosophically disillusioned	o. Firing people
16. Kinetic kill vehicle	p. Nuclear war

Answers to the Doublespeak of the Would-be Leader

1. Don't look a gift horse in the mouth.
2. Haste makes waste.
3. Don't cross the bridge until you come to it.
4. Don't cut off your nose to spite your face.
5. Don't put all your eggs in one basket.
6. Brevity is the soul of wit.

1. g
2. l
3. b
4. m
5. j
6. c
7. o
8. h
9. n
10. p
11. f
12. e
13. d
14. a
15. i
16. k

Remember:

Winston Churchill asserted, "Big men use little words." When we think of leaders who have inspired us, we usually find that they were sharing strong beliefs with very basic words.

Using humor appropriately is part of effective communication, telling a personal story of error or humor that makes you one of the group is a great icebreaker.

Team Creativity Exercise 2

Practice Panic: The A-B-Cs

Every practice has one of those days when something unexpected causes a panic; every person is tempted to make knee-jerk reactions. It only takes one sane mind to pull out the candy tin with the cards and dice and say, "Let's do the A-B-Cs."

Objective

Many of us have done it for fun, so let's use it for practice creativity: random sequence associations. The idea is to bring together different thoughts in new associations. The only tools you need to use are 3×5-inch index cards and three dice, each a different color.

Building the Candy Tin Box

Just use a tin box, or a cigar box, or something that has a unique appearance so it does not get lost in the practice clutter. Keep it in the pharmacy or lab (thus the need for the stain resistance of a metal box). The box only needs to be large enough to hold some 3×5-inch index cards and three dice. Go find three dice, each a different color, and put them in the box and then build the basic theme cards.

The theme cards are practice specific. They represent areas of relationships. Ideas include but are not limited to

- Community needs
- Client perceptions
- Patient needs
- Staff desires
- Doctor preferences
- Resources available
- Services and products
- Success scoring

The theme cards can be adjusted (e.g., new ones added) for each panic, but remember, each card represents a major area of idea exploration, so keep the topic general enough to allow at least six subcategories for each theme card. When in a panic, pull out the theme cards, see if a new theme card needs to be introduced based on the panic of the moment, and pick only three of the theme cards—these will become columns A, B, and C.

After selecting the three theme cards and assigning the appropriate colored dice and column position (it does not matter in what order), create six options for each of the relationship areas. This is done by calling together the team members and having everyone offer ideas for the columns. The final three-column brain-storm product may appear as follows:

<u>**Community Needs**</u> *<u>red dice</u>*	<u>**Resources Available**</u> *<u>white dice</u>*	<u>**Success Scoring**</u> *<u>blue dice</u>*
1. morning drop-off	1. colleagues	1. staff pride
2. economic services	2. money	2. media accolade
3. teenager help	3. VIN @ aol.com	3. new clients
4. easier access	4. time	4. dollars
5. exotic care	5. paper	5. white board hash marks
6. yuppy harmony	6. muscles	6. client returns

Now it is time to let the dice do the walkin' so your team can do the talkin'. Roll the three dice and let them associate a trio of words. What thoughts do the new linkages inspire from the team? Let it be fun and let the ideas flow. When the well runs dry, toss the dice again. With each toss of the dice, new opportunities will emerge. If three tosses of the dice fail to elicit any good ideas, reshuffle the theme cards and repeat the process.

These associations and ideas are starting stimuli, no more, but no less. Often, they should not be taken literally. Be careful: if the group is made up of highly structured, tight-lipped, process-oriented players, the results may be more frustrating than rewarding for them until they learn to loosen up *and smile*.

The A-B-Cs in Action

In one case, a practice was panicked when Ms. Rossi threatened a hate campaign because of a large bill. We rolled the dice and got 3-4-1, and if we had the above cards, that would have meant: *teenager help–time–staff pride*. What could this do for us with Ms. Rossi? Was she a source for teenager part-time help, or was she active in Exploring and needed our help? Was there a need to give her more time to vent, or did we keep her too long without giving her adequate one-on-one time? If her daughter took a position as a weekend bather, would her pride show, or did our staff stress give the wrong message, rather than pride in what we had done?

We had the attending doctor call Ms. Rossi and ask for some *time* to better understand her concerns. We asked her, "What can we do to make it right?" and shared our concern about keeping our clients happy—*we let our pride show!* We never found the teen linkage, but that was okay.

Team Creativity Exercise 3
Break the Law

Paradigms (more than just two thin 10 cent pieces) abound in veterinary medicine. We have been limited by years of education (the best solution of the moment becoming the *only* alternative), practice acts, federal regulations, and our own life experiences and biases. The fact is, what we think may not necessarily be so. ...

Objective

To break the law, we must first consider a task in terms of perceived limitations, cliches, regulations, popular opinions, and traditions. Then we must examine what happens if we ignore, circumvent, or redefine the intent of those limitations. What happens when the thou shalt nots are removed from the thought process?

Get Calibrated to Get Started

Look at some of the Great Laws we have encountered on the way to developing our own veterinary practice:

- Only the best get into veterinary school.
- The world is flat.
- Anyone can be a receptionist.
- The sun rotates around the earth.
- Nice guys finish last.
- Chows are cute and cuddly dogs.
- Corporate sponsorship of practices will kill this profession.
- Business owners get to set their own hours.
- All fruit drinks are shades of yellow, orange, or red.

Now look at your task. List the laws, regulations, constraining perceptions, and practice traditions that control the how, when, where, what, and resources. Now next to each law, twist the "shall not" into "thou shall" that proves the law wrong. Start breaking laws three at a time; make violations the rule of your thought process—never stay linear. Heck, be a rebel and find a way to violate all of them at once. Thumb your nose at those who say, "It can't be done," and prove that *the usual can be done in an unusual way and the unusual can be done as if it were usual.*

Now consider the thought process that was used—feel the havoc in your gut. This is called change. Luck is not magic; it is simply the result of the practice being prepared to grab opportunity as it passes by the front door. By changing the rules, where do the consequence take you? How does it change the situation? In what way does it liberate the team?

Breaking the Examination Room Law

For years, people argued about 15-minute, versus 20-minute, versus 30-minute appointments in companion animal practice. In this text, I introduced a variable configuration, a 10-minute, out-of-sync, high-density scheduling system using an outpatient nurse technician assigned to a doctor to schedule two exam rooms concurrently. This is a wonderful example of breaking the practice paradigm of linear thinking and how to make many practitioners very uncomfortable. Look at what else can be done to break the rules:

- We schedule examination rooms rather than doctors.
- We call technicians "nurses" because clients understand the term.
- The practice controls client access via the receptionists.
- We do 19 patients in four hours, a 100 percent increase in doctor usage.
- Inpatient teams handle walk-ins and emergencies.
- We use 10-minute slots for suture removals and rechecks.
- We use 20-minute slots for outpatient sick call and annual consultations.
- We use 30-minute slots for new clients and exotics.
- We give new graduates extra time on *every* appointment.

Many veterinarians will say, "This is not new; we do it every Saturday." To this I reply, "Why did you not learn from your own experience and do it all week?" Why are double standards okay, but change resisted? Why do some rules and laws apply at all times, and others selectively, sometimes, it appears, just to frustrate the practice team? Law breakers need to have a spiritual basis of thought.

Once laws are written on paper, alternatives begin to appear, some appropriate, some fattening, and some illegal. The core values of the practice cannot be violated, but the philosophy or mission may need redefinition. The break the law process will solidify the practice core values and will also slay the dragons threatening to eat the team's creative juices.

Team Creativity Exercise 4
The Practice Puzzle

In healthcare promotions, we don't "sell" things to the clients, we "allow them to buy" based on their perceived needs and desires. Some clients hate to buy but far more hate to be sold something. What we market in healthcare delivery is peace of mind. For instance:

- They don't sell coal—they sell warmth.
- They don't sell glasses—they sell vision.
- We don't sell preanesthetic labs—we sell patient safety.
- They don't sell clothes—they sell a new image.
- They don't sell movies—they sell entertainment.
- We don't sell dentistries—we sell less bad breath.
- We don't buy circus tickets—we buy thrills.
- We don't sell discount coupons—please—ever!

Objective

The practice puzzle is to identify what is really being offered, so it forces your team to center on the feelings of your clients. You must think more about the intangibles, the implications of your healthcare process, and less about the task itself. You must focus on hopes, emotions, and client-centered benefits and go past that mission statement to the core of your practice philosophy.

How to Make It Occur

You should already have defined your mission and maybe even the practice philosophy or core values of the practice. Ensure everyone keeps these in mind when you play Practice Puzzle. Bring the staff together and form everyone into a circle—doctors too. Now as a team, define what you are trying to accomplish with one specific program. What are you trying to change? Who do you want to listen? What is the message? Now complete the following two statements:

- We don't sell (task in concrete, traditional terms)
- We let them buy (abstract sensation or emotion)

Have each team member complete the above statement as quickly as possible. You are looking for the soft stuff the clients are made of, not technical jargon. Look at the consequences, secondary benefits, emotions, gut instincts, perceptions, attitudes, and intuitions that drive day-by-day animal stewardship.

After the cycle has been done a couple of times around the staff ring, post the list of responses on the staff bulletin board and let it mature. Each staff member should look at the blanks that have been completed and assess why the emotion was important to some person in the staff ring. Set aside the value judgements and try to understand why each blank was filled in as it was.

Use each statement to develop narratives for client discussion. Use it as a starting point for new ways to state patient or practice needs as well as new ways to offer practice programs. Each statement is an opportunity to sell peace of mind to a client. Consider each a challenge to find a new direction or perspective to better become an advocate of our patient or professional ethics. Look for shortfalls to support and strengths to share with others.

- We don't sell vaccines—we sell protection.
- We don't sell vaccines—we let clients buy protection.
- We don't sell vaccines—we let clients buy protection for their animals.
- We don't sell vaccines—we let clients buy protection for their families.
- We don't sell vaccines—we let clients buy freedom from anguish.
- We don't sell vaccines—we let clients buy compliance to the law.
- We don't sell vaccines—we let clients select disease reduction.
- We don't sell vaccines—we let clients buy peace of mind.

And it can continue ... and it should. The staff members need to rise to the occasion and develop their own beliefs and positions.

Team Creativity Exercise 5
Realm of Resource Research

The need for stimuli is a constant in veterinary practice, and great ideas come from unlikely sources. This exercise requires using lateral paraprofessional journals and references, like *Better Homes and Garden, Cat Fancy, JCPenney Catalog, Dog Fancy, Cosmopolitan, Pet Store News, Ladies Home Journal, Birds of PanAmerica, Time, Quarter Horse Journal,* Dr. Seuss's books, *Dairy Herdsman,* or similar publications.

Objective

Realm of resource research is a jump start, a way to leave the linear tracks of veterinary medical thought and start looking at the perspectives of the client. This uses the printed word to jar staff members out of routine thinking and to expand the implications of whatever task they have at hand.

Getting It Done

Stack the publications on a coffee table; you need at least a dozen representing over half-a-dozen different titles (for different trains of thought/different editorial perspectives). It really does not matter what the date is: some older ones are now revolutionary and have improved with age. Each person gets a pillow and sits on the floor around the table. Come well stocked with coffee, Mountain Dew, tea, Coke, and other caffeine-fix sources. Start the background music (not the clinical elevator music), preferably stuff not usually listened to by the team, like Disney songs, the theme from *Rocky,* or other motivational music.

Now, randomly insert an index card somewhere in the pages of at least six of the publications. If you have trouble doing this, give each person three index cards and have each person insert them into publications (no peeking at where). At this point, open to an index card and let your eyes do the walking—look at the page as a complex set of hints and ideas, waiting to be understood. Use the images and concepts as stimuli.

■ Why was the editor committed to putting this article/picture in the publication?
■ What emotions has the author appealed to in the article?
■ If there is a picture, create a new caption!
■ If this was yours, how would you use it in your neighborhood?
■ What functions, or actions, could be this be used for?
■ How does this relate to the challenge of the moment?
■ Uh, what's up doc?

The best method is for each person to select something, show it to the group, and relate his/her first thought about it. The person across offers his/her perception, and then the person across from him/her does the same. Do not overassess or overthink; use the first impression and build on it with others if you think it is a great idea. Let the mind froggy (hop from point to point without clear direction). As the pace slackens, consume some more caffeine and then restart the process with another publication. Play some other music to excite the senses. Then restart the process with more caffeine and another publication. Play some other music.

Does This Really Work?

We were building our office complex (yes, Mabel, we do construction as well as consultation) and fixing a plumbing leak, from the leasehold unit next door, that had flooded our bathroom (my associate Phil is really a Master Plumber). We had not completed the task, but we had stopped the leak and were taking a break; we were drinking our caffeine fix and talking about the final office configuration. We had opened up some office design and supply catalogs to look at cabinets and other data retrieval systems.

I saw a cabinet system that was displayed as a built-in. We had already used my desk as a built-in, with an under-the-top bookcase on both sides, one in my office and one on the other side of the wall in the adjoining office. The wall above the desk was just a glass window between the offices. This system was the result of a custom design brainstorm, and we were very proud of it. But the built-in office supply cabinet caught my eye—it was tall and narrow. It was about as wide as the hole we had cut into the plumbing wall to fix the leak. I showed Phil, and a light appeared in his eye. We walked to the bath and looked at the 1-foot square low on the wall and had the following discussion:

- ■ "We can extend this hole upward 5 feet."
- ■ "We can make it the full width between two studs."
- ■ "We can build a cabinet and slip it into the wall."
- ■ "We can bolt the cabinet to the studs so it is removable if another leak occurs."
- ■ "We can use simple framing around the hole and not worry about finishing the drywall at the hole."

We now have a built-in bathroom supply cabinet in the rest room, and many people don't even notice the built-in appearance until we mention it. The synergy system does work, if you look beyond the obvious.

Team Creativity Exercise 6
The Staff Members Are Your Gems

There are precious gems and semiprecious gems, never bad gems.

In my seminars, I talk about the difference between a real diamond and a synthetic one (cubic zirconium). The point is that real diamonds have flaws while the fakes are perfect; we even name diamonds for their flaws (Pink Panther, Star of India, etc.). It is our flaws that make us people and are why we must build jobs around a person's strengths rather than pounding the person into a specific size "job hole." This exercise allows us to classify the gems in your practice. I don't know its origin; I ran across it at a CE course at ACHE, where the seminar leader did not know its origin either, but regardless, it is an effective tool. I've named it the Gem Score.

It is a tool, not an end result nor a tablet to be inscribed on the mountain and brought down to the masses. The bottom line is this: the following is simply a game to discover the value of the gems in your practice. Some are precious, and others are semiprecious, but it is very unlikely that you have cubic zirconiums— we don't pay enough to have people stick with us just for the pleasure of long days, nasty clients, and a grouchy doctor. The scoring system is not scientifically sound; it is designed to start discussions. The discussions start where most problems stop, when something must be *proven, built,* or *found.* The summaries are not designed to provide comprehensive profiles, but they are designed to provide a starting point for exploration into the value of the gems in your practice—the *provers, builders,* and *finders.*

Now go and have fun, and if you don't plan to have fun, you need to read *Building the Successful Veterinary Practice: Leadership Tools.* Leaders know how to have fun, since it balances the dedication and commitment associated with the hard-working practice. Now go, have fun, smile, and enjoy the sparkling gems in your life.

The Gem Score

This survey is environmentally dependent, so stay focused on the practice setting rather than home, church, sports, or elsewhere. It provides some insight, so take it with a song in your heart; you will not die from the results, since the results are neither right nor wrong—they are only the total of your answers. This survey looks at the feelings you have about yourself. If you feel closer to one trait than another, that is okay; it is expected. If you are both, or neither, that is okay; circle a number in the center. Use any number you feel like, but circle *only* one number for each question.

Do you see yourself as more

1. Sophisticated   Down-to-Earth
   0   1   2   3   4   5   6   7   8   9   10
2. Outgoing   Shy
   0   1   2   3   4   5   6   7   8   9   10
3. Saver   Spender
   0   1   2   3   4   5   6   7   8   9   10
4. Expect the Best   Expect the Worse
   0   1   2   3   4   5   6   7   8   9   10
5. Critical   Forgiving
   0   1   2   3   4   5   6   7   8   9   10
6. Easygoing   Intense
   0   1   2   3   4   5   6   7   8   9   10
7. Boring   Exciting
   0   1   2   3   4   5   6   7   8   9   10
8. Cautious   Adventurous
   0   1   2   3   4   5   6   7   8   9   10
9. Humorous   Serious
   0   1   2   3   4   5   6   7   8   9   10
10. Predictable   Spontaneous
   0   1   2   3   4   5   6   7   8   9   10

Now that you are done, it's time for some addition. First, please transfer your scores to the following ... without changing or brooding.

Add the Following Scores

Number from # 1   _____
Number from # 3   _____
Number from # 5   _____
Number from # 7   _____
Number from # 8   _____
Number from # 10 _____

Add the Following Scores

Number from # 2   _____
Number from # 4   _____
Number from # 6   _____
Number from # 9   _____

SUBTOTAL A =   _____

SUBTOTAL B =   _____

(40 + Subtotal A) - Subtotal B = _____ = Gem Score

There are no right or wrong Gem Scores. Each has its own mix of strengths and opportunities (the opposite of strength is weakness and the opposite of opportunity is threat, but we will stay positive, right? Right!). In an ideal group, there will be a perfect mix of perfect people—but that is not a veterinary practice, so do not hold your breath. People come in a rainbow of traits, but this exercise focuses on only three (and it doesn't matter if you are on the cusp):

Prove It: shoulder to the wheel, eye on the road, feet on the ground—practical, tactical, and focused solidly on the reality of today.

Build It: everything has a middle ground, each person has a point—synthesizers, peacemakers, compromisers, and focused on making most people feel good.

Find It: tomorrow is always the opportunity, it will be better, the dream makes the problem no big deal—new ideas, change, and continual improvement replaces the status quo.

The Gem Score ranges from 0, the hardest of the hard, the realist of renown, all the way to 100, the ultimate starry-eyed dreamer. The score is as accurate as the mind-set you had when you completed the exercise or as accurate as the mind-set of the other person looking at the score. It doesn't matter. As you learned in school, "Man classifies; Mother Nature just occurs." Just use the following definitions as milestones on the road to releasing the power of the team.

Prove It (0 to 56)
A practical person, just like *over half* of corporate America. The talent for taking an idea and exploiting it has made Prove It folk famous. They approach the world as a balance between positives and negatives and are skilled at spotting bumps in the road, snags in the river, hurdles on the track, and land mines in the process. They accept their brilliance well and see themselves as a bit smarter than the average Joe. For all of this, their great ideas are usually expansions of others, reworkings of existing situations or things to better tackle the reality of the day.

Make It Happen: To get their creative juices flowing, allow these folk to be incremental. Give them a starting point and a clear definition of the need; let them see it, feel it, and smell it. They are at their best when they are reacting to their thoughts.

Build It (57–67)
A broad view expert, looking at all features with an equal concern for the other person's perspective. This is the person who spans the space between the realist and the dreamer who live at the extremes of the Gem Scores. These are the famous orchestrators of harmony, the mediators, and the frustrating middle roaders who don't think it is important to take a stand at the expense of another. This ringleader often sees the values of ideas better than those presenting

them. Ambidexterity is their forte! They can take the raw thoughts of others and give them depth and perspective that most all can rally around.

Make It Happen: Lubricate this person's thinking by increasing the flow of ideas between the two poles. Ask him/her to expand and elaborate on a concept, never to evaluate. Build It folk will be the ones who nurture that acorn into a mighty oak.

Find It (68–100)

These folk have vision down pat. They try to stay off the beaten path so they can more easily find the opportunity. The blank page is a friend, asking for help. These folk excel without structure and are stressed with protocols and process, so let them have the freedom to walk in the woods and play in the sandbox. No wonder they compose only about 15 percent of corporate America.

Make It Happen: Become a Trekkie—ask them to go where no person has gone before. These will be the catalysts of new ideas, the spark plugs. When the environment allows, they will make leaps of faith and hurtle ideas through time and space faster than through the wormhole of Deep Space Nine.

How to Nurture the Creative Process of Gem Score Individuals

Provers

Nike's slogan will help—Just do it! To break the ice, make them play in a childlike way. If necessary, provide a field trip to a preschool for at least an hour of crawling and playing with the kids. Their eye for flaws can be a drawback, so repeat the theme of *The Little Engine That Could*. Put them into an unfamiliar environment that requires sensory commitments; tell them to hit the bricks, survey the mall, walk the woods, and *listen, listen, listen* to others. When you throw them out of their safe environment, nurture them to open up about their new feelings, and they will help make things happen.

Builders

Since these people always look for the good of both sides, beware of complacency. They straddle the fence and never feel the rail themselves; forward progress is not on their agenda. These traits makes the builders good facilitators, when tasked and prodded. Have them play for the rebound off the boards, ask for the flip side of a concept, or even task them to lead an exploration of the downside of an upbeat idea or the upside of a doom and gloom discussion. They need to have a conflict to excel, so asking them to accept the role of devil's advocate for both sides would be a great benefit to the creative process.

Finders

The secret here is to get others to listen and nurture—they need no help dreaming of what could be. Most will ask them to prove their point (remember the Prove It group is in the majority), and this will shut down the process. Use the builders to help model the idea; prototypes built by others will assist the process. Since these folk will often work on many levels simultaneously, multiple scribes may be needed, just to keep up and sort the flow. Narrowing the focus once into the process will help these players stay in the game. Use the people-oriented feelings of the finders to remind the group of the value of the provers—do not let anyone reject their ideas or refuse to listen ... others are the key to changing the ideas of finders into reality.

Team Creativity Exercise 7
Guinness—The Book, Not the Stout

This is a fast-paced, highly targeted, focusing project. It is a shortcut to locating and explaining your advantages and your assets, and it helps the team focus its energy on the bright points of the practice day.

Objective

You want to isolate one or two facets of a practice task that could shine brighter, and cause more pride, in the eyes of people outside the practice. This exercise is a fast-track method in establishing

- A common hot button of pride
- An emerging professional/technical opportunity
- A service no one has offered to the community before
- An opportunity for practice growth (increasing return rates or new clients)
- A way to remedy a perceived shortfall in community veterinary services
- An area of the practice that can produce more net
- A clear point of difference between your practice and others in the area

Doing It

Get a *Guinness Book of World Records*—the unabridged size; it is a great source of creative ideas. Essentially, you want your practice to achieve a new record in veterinary healthcare delivery in the community. You must find that gee whiz feature and corner that accolade—but how do you select one?

Start with areas that the team wants to research, areas it wants to push, poke, and explore. Be trivial in the exploration, since it is *breadth* that is needed during the research phase, *not depth*. Follow your instincts, not your logic; expand on your feelings, not on dollars. Cover all the foothills and get ready to make them mountains. Don't start to climb just a single mountaintop—it is likely that everyone has already seen that one!

Give each brainstormed advantage or asset a special practice award, such as Most Caring, Most Feline Friendly, Most Unlike Us, Most Exciting, Most Radical, Most Likely to Make Competitors Worry, Least Complex, Biggest Boss Surprise, Most Appealing to Seniors, or Most Likely to Affect the Net. Be generous in the development of awards; make sure every awarded aspect qualifies the practice or individual for Guinness-level recognition.

Team Creativity Exercise 8
Mind-Mapping Webs

Every thought process is a systematic selection of ideas, but mind mapping does not involve selection. It is an expansion of ideas. Some say Tony Buzan started it, but since most lawyers have been taught it, that is suspect. Regardless, it is a system of recording free association and making the chaos of free thought work for you and your practice team.

Objective

Take a single task or thought and make it bulge, blossom, and network with other thoughts. Mind mapping is a way to invent alternatives to challenges and to evolve solutions from the chaos of the human mind. In fact, it is designed to prevent single-thought threads and horse blinders from ruling your life.

The Old Way

When you were young, you scribbled, and then you went to school and became organized. Your teachers taught you to think in a linear fashion. In fact, they taught you to outline before you got out of grade school to emphasize the importance of linear thinking:

A. Challenge
  1. Big
  2. Medium
  3. Small
B. Problem
  1. Nice
  2. Bad

Even though linear thinking greatly limits people's approach to real-life problems, current public education is based on eliminating the alternatives and ensuring you have only the one best answer to the problem of the moment (and hence, multiple-choice questions were born).

Weaving the Web

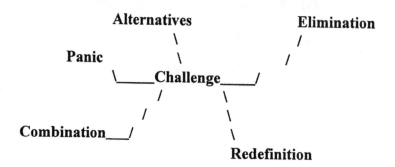

Get a BIG sheet of paper—the bigger the better. Then clearly define the task, the objective, the central challenge (often this is a who, what, where, when, or why). Write it in the center of the sheet of paper and draw a parallelogram, pentagon, or hexagon around it (if you use a bold color marker, all the better). At each corner, come up with a major area for exploration and draw a line outward from that corner and write down the new major area. As with Buzan's mind mapping, the thought process is now shown in two dimensions, and this generally creates a messy, free-form, dynamic method of writing thoughts on paper.

This process starts to unleash the imagination. Push yourself by expanding each thought four or five ways—never limit yourself to linear thinking in this process. As you free-associate outward, spokes of ideas are formed, and the farther from the center you get, the more the opportunities for further expansion will occur. The ideas for the spokes will also deviate farther from reality as you know it and will more closely approach the new and different for the practice. If needed, stimulate the thought process by reviewing picture-heavy magazines and coffee-table books, with color pictures, to expand the spectrum of thought. Let the juices flow!

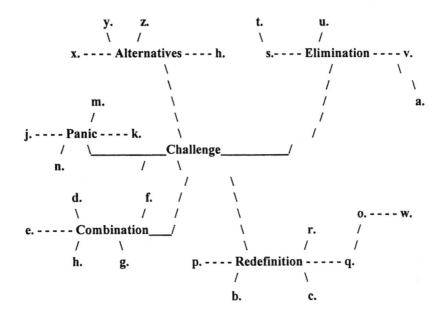

Review the map and put geometric figures around the great ideas that deserve further development. If your team is in the groove, you will likely use different color markers so that new colors and shapes are related to great new ideas. Draw stars, use exclamation points, and let the excitement begin!